HANDBOOK OF
Orthopaedic
Rehabilitation

D0027122

HANDBOOK OF
Orthopaedic
Rehabilitation

EDITOR

S. BRENT BROTZMAN, MD

Staff Orthopaedic Surgeon
  Spohn Hospital;
Chief of Foot and Ankle Service
  Orthopaedic Surgery and Sports Medicine Associates
Corpus Christi, Texas

with 176 illustrations

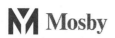 Mosby

St. Louis   Baltimore   Boston
Carlsbad   Chicago   Naples   New York   Philadelphia   Portland
London   Madrid   Mexico City   Singapore   Sydney   Tokyo   Toronto   Wiesbaden

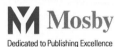

Mosby

Dedicated to Publishing Excellence

A Times Mirror Company

Publisher: Anne S. Patterson
Editor: Kathryn H. Falk
Developmental Editor: Carolyn Malik
Project Manager: John Rogers
Production Editor: Cheryl Abbott Bozzay
Designer: Renée Duenow
Manufacturing Supervisor: Linda Ierardi

Printed in the United States of America
Composition by Clarinda Company
Printing/binding by RR Donnelley & Sons, Company

Mosby–Year Book, Inc.
11830 Westline Industrial Drive
St. Louis, Missouri 63146

Library of Congress Cataloging in Publication Data

Handbook of orthopaedic rehabilitation / S. Brent Brotzman, editor.
    p.   cm.
    Includes index.
    ISBN 0-8151-1102-9
    1. Physically handicapped—Rehabilitation—Handbooks, manuals, etc. 2. Orthopedics—Handbooks, manuals, etc. I. Brotzman, S. Brent.
    [DNLM: 1. Orthopedics—methods—handbooks. 2. Rehabilitation--standards—handbooks. WE 39 H2365 1995]
RD799.H36   1995
617.3—dc20
DNLM/DLC
for Library of Congress   95-42301
                            CIP

97 98 99 00 / 9 8 7 6 5 4 3 2

Contributing Authors

KELLY AKIN, PT
Staff Physical Therapist
    Physical Therapy Department
    Campbell Clinic
Memphis, Tennessee

JAMES R. ANDREWS, MD
Clinical Professor of Orthopaedics and Sports Medicine
    University of Virginia School of Medicine;
Clinical Professor, Department of Orthopaedic Surgery
    University of Kentucky Medical Center;
Medical Director, American Sports Medicine Institute
    Birmingham, Alabama

MARYLYLE BOOLOS, PT, AT, C
Rehabilitation Hospital of the Mid-South
Memphis, Tennessee

JILL BRASEL, PT
Clinical Coordinator
    Physical Therapy Department
    Campbell Clinic
Memphis, Tennessee

S. BRENT BROTZMAN, MD
Staff Orthopaedic Surgeon
    Spohn Hospital;
Chief of Foot and Ankle Service
    Orthopaedic Surgery and Sports Medicine Associates
Corpus Christi, Texas

JAMES H. CALANDRUCCIO, MD
Instructor
    University of Tennessee–Campbell Clinic
    Department of Orthopaedic Surgery;
Staff Orthopaedic Surgeon
    Campbell Clinic
Memphis, Tennessee

HUGH U. CAMERON, MB, CHB, FRCS(C), FAAOS
Associate Professor
  Departments of Surgery, Pathology, and Engineering
  University of Toronto;
Staff Orthopaedic Surgeon
  Orthopaedic and Arthritic Hospital
Toronto, Canada

DAVID GROH, PT
Staff Physical Therapist
  HealthSouth Sports Medicine and Rehabilitation Center
Birmingham, Alabama

PENNY HEAD, PT, AT, C
Sports Medicine Coordinator
  Physical Therapy Department
  Campbell Clinic
Memphis, Tennessee

FRANK W. JOBE, MD
Associate, Kerlan–Jobe Clinic;
Clinical Professor, Department of Orthopaedics
  University of Southern California School of Medicine;
Orthopaedic Consultant
  Los Angeles Dodgers
  PGA Tour
  Senior PGA Tour
Los Angeles, California

MARK T. JOBE, MD
Assistant Professor
  University of Tennessee–Campbell Clinic
  Department of Orthopaedic Surgery;
Staff Orthopaedic Surgeon
  Campbell Clinic
Memphis, Tennessee

ANA K. PALMIERI, MD
Orthopaedic Resident
  University of Tennessee–Campbell Clinic
  Department of Orthopaedic Surgery
Memphis, Tennessee

THOMAS A. RUSSELL, MD
Associate Professor
 University of Tennessee–Campbell Clinic
 Department of Orthopaedic Surgery;
Russell Orthopaedic Center;
Staff Orthopaedic Surgeon
 Methodist Hospital
Memphis, Tennessee

DIANE MOYNE SCHWAB, MS, PT
Champion Rehabilitation
San Diego, California

ARTHUR H. WHITE, MD
Medical Director
 SpineCare Medical Group;
Medical Director
 San Francisco Spine Institute;
Past President, North American Spine Society
San Francisco, California

KEVIN E. WILK, PT
National Director, Research and Clinical Education
 HealthSouth Rehabilitation Corporation;
Associate Clinical Director
 HealthSouth Rehabilitation Center;
Director of Rehabilitative Research
 American Sports Medicine Institute
Birmingham;
Adjunct Assistant Professor
 Marquette University
 Programs in Physician Therapy
Milwaukee, Wisconsin

To my loving wife
Cynthia
whose patience and understanding
throughout the long process
have provided inspiration and encouragement,
and to my parents,
whose love and sacrifice over the years
have given me countless opportunities.

Preface

Although the literature describing orthopaedic surgical techniques and acute fracture care is sound and comprehensive, there is relatively little easily-referenced information concerning postoperative or postfracture rehabilitation. This void persisted despite the fact that rehabilitation therapy may have as much or more effect on long-term results than the initial treatment of an injury or condition. A technically superb surgical result may be compromised by improper postoperative rehabilitation techniques that allow scar formation, stiffness, rupture of incompletely healed tissue, or loss of function.

This handbook is designed to give the reader well-established rehabilitation protocols used by leading orthopaedic surgeons and therapists in specific specialty areas. These protocols are *not* intended to be used with a cookbook approach that would fit every possible situation or patient; but they are designed to give the reader a framework on which individualized programs can be built. Additional protocols on conditions covered in this handbook and on some conditions not covered here, as well as extensive rehabilitation rationale, background information, and bibliographies may be found in the larger textbook, *Clinical Orthopaedic Rehabilitation*. The textbook also contains rehabilitation information for low back disorders, pediatric fractures, and reflex sympathetic dystrophy; and it covers the use of foot orthoses.

Many existing rehabilitation protocols are empirically based and have been shaped by years of "trial and error" in large numbers of patients. Changes in rehabilitation approaches may be indicated in the future by the results of clinical research and biomechanical studies. At present, however, the principles outlined in this text are those accepted by most orthopaedic surgeons and therapists.

It is hoped that this handbook will provide physicians and therapists with a concise, easy-to-use guide for formulating rehabilitation protocols that will best serve their patients.

Acknowledgements

I would like to acknowledge the valuable contributions of a number of people who made this book possible. First, my thanks to all of the surgeons and therapists who were kind enough to invest the time and effort required to share their expertise. Thanks also to the Campbell Foundation crew: to Kay Daugherty for her editing skills, to Joan Crowson for her help in obtaining both obvious and obscure references, and to Linda Jones for her assistance in manuscript preparation. My special thanks to the staff of the Campbell Clinic for their generous and unfailing willingness to answer questions, give advice, and provide encouragement.

Of course, this text would not have been possible without the assistance and encouragement of all the staff at Mosby–Year Book. My thanks to all who believed the work was worthwhile and patiently guided a first-time author.

S. Brent Brotzman

Contents

HANDBOOK OF
Orthopaedic
Rehabilitation

CHAPTER ONE

Rehabilitation of the Hand and Wrist

JAMES H. CALANDRUCCIO, MD
MARK T. JOBE, MD
KELLY AKIN, PT

Many of the rehabilitation protocols in this chapter are taken from *Diagnosis and Treatment Manual for Physicians and Therapists* by Nancy Cannon, OTR. These protocols are designated by an asterisk. We highly recommend this manual as a detailed reference text for hand therapy.

Flexor Tendon Injuries
REHABILITATION RATIONALE AND BASIC PRINCIPLES

Timing
The timing of flexor tendon repair influences the rehabilitation and outcome of flexor tendon injuries.
- *Primary repair* is performed within the first 12 to 24 hours after injury.
- *Delayed primary repair* is performed within the first 10 days after injury.

  ■ If primary repair is not performed, delayed primary repair should be performed as soon as there is evidence of wound healing without infection.
- *Secondary repair* is performed more than 10 to 14 days after injury.
- *Late secondary repair* is performed more than 4 weeks after injury.

After 4 weeks, it is extremely difficult to deliver the flexor tendon through the digital sheath, which usually becomes extensively scarred. If the sheath is not scarred or destroyed, single-stage tendon grafting, direct repair, or tendon transfer may be performed. If extensive disturbance and scarring has occurred, two-stage tendon grafting with a Hunter rod technique should be used.

Anatomy
The anatomic zone of injury of the flexor tendons influences the outcome and rehabilitation of these injuries. The hand is divided into five distinct flexor zones.
- Zone 1—from the insertion of the profundus tendon at the distal phalanx to just distal to the insertion of the sublimis.
- Zone 2—Bunnell's "no-man's land"—the critical area of pulleys between the insertion of the sublimis and the distal palmar crease.

Text and illustrations in this chapter marked with an asterisk (*) are modified from or redrawn from Cannon NM: *Diagnosis and treatment manual for physicians and therapists,* ed 3, 1991, The Hand Rehabilitation Center of Indiana, PC.

- Zone 3—"area of lumbrical origin"—from the beginning of the pulleys (A1) to the distal margin of the transverse carpal ligament.
- Zone 4—area covered by the transverse carpal ligament.
- Zone 5—area proximal to the transverse carpal ligament.

■ *As a rule, repairs to tendons injured outside the flexor sheath have much better results than repairs to tendons injured inside the sheath (zone 2).*

Rehabilitation

The rehabilitation protocol chosen for a patient depends on the *timing* of the repair (delayed primary or secondary), the *location* of the injury (zones 1 through 5), and the *compliance* of the patient (early mobilization for compliant patients or delayed mobilization for noncompliant patients and children younger than 7 years of age).

■ *The two most frequent causes for failure of primary tendon repairs are formation of adhesions and rupture of the repaired tendon, respectively.*

REHABILITATION PROTOCOL

Immediate (or Delayed Primary) Repair of Injury in Zone 1, 2, or 3: Modified Duran Protocol*

Prerequisites: compliant patient
clean or healed wound
repair within 14 days of injury

1 to 3 days

- Remove bulky compressive dressing and apply light compressive dressing.
- Digital level fingersocks or coban are utilized for edema control.
- Fit dorsal blocking splint (DBS) to wrist and digits for continual wear with following positions:
  Wrist—20 degrees of flexion.
  Metacarpophalangeal (MCP) joints—50 degrees of flexion.
  Distal interphalangeal (DIP) and proximal interphalangeal (PIP) joints—full extension.

- Initiate controlled passive mobilization exercises, including passive flexion/extension exercises to DIP and PIP joints individually.
- Composite passive flexion/extension exercises to MCP, PIP, DIP joints of digits (modified Duran program). Active extension should be within the restraints of DBS. If full passive flexion is not obtained, the patient may begin prolonged flexion stretching with Coban or taping.
- 8 repetitions each of isolated passive flexion/extension exercises of the MCP, PIP, and DIP within the DBS (Figs. 1-1, 1-2, and 1-3).

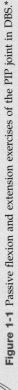

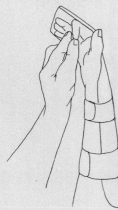

Figure 1-1 Passive flexion and extension exercises of the PIP joint in DBS.*

Figure 1-2 Passive flexion and extension exercises of the DIP joint in DBS.*

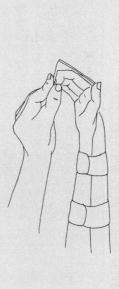

Figure 1-3 Combined passive flexion and extension exercises of the MCP, PIP, and DIP joints.*

Continued

REHABILITATION PROTOCOL—cont'd

Immediate (or Delayed Primary) Repair of Injury in Zone 1, 2, or 3: Modified Duran Protocol*

4.5 weeks	• Continue the exercises and begin active ROM for fingers and wrist flexion, allowing active wrist extension to neutral or 0 degrees of extension only. • Patients should perform hourly exercises with the splint removed, including composite fist, wrist flexion and extension to neutral, composite finger flexion with the wrist immobilized (Fig. 1-4). • Have patient perform fist to hook fist (intrinsic minus position) exercise to extended fingers (Fig. 1-5). • Watch for PIP flexion contractures. If an extension lag is present, add protected passive extension of PIP joint with MCP held in flexion—this should be performed only by reliable patients or therapists. The PIP joint should be blocked to
	30 degrees of flexion for 3 weeks if a concomitant distal nerve repair is performed. • Patients may reach a plateau in ROM 2 months after surgery; however, maximal motion is usually achieved by 3 months after surgery.
5 weeks	• FES (functional electrical stimulation) may be used to improve tendon excursion. Consider the patient's quality of primary repair, the nature of the injury, and the medical history before initiating FES.
5.5 weeks	• Add blocking exercises for PIP and DIP joints to previous home program. • Discontinue DBS.

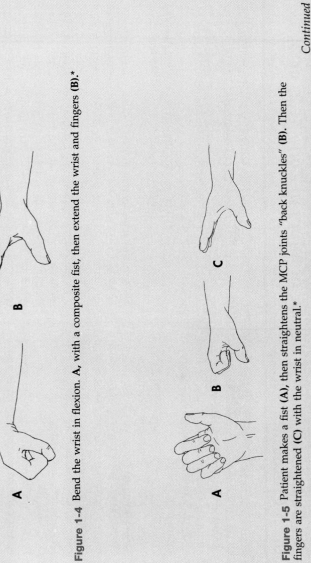

Figure 1-4 Bend the wrist in flexion. **A**, with a composite fist, then extend the wrist and fingers **(B)**.*

Figure 1-5 Patient makes a fist **(A)**, then straightens the MCP joints "back knuckles" **(B)**. Then the fingers are straightened **(C)** with the wrist in neutral.*

Continued

REHABILITATION PROTOCOL—cont'd

Immediate (or Delayed Primary) Repair of Injury in Zone 1, 2, or 3: Modified Duran Protocol*

5.5 weeks—cont'd	• Focus should be on gaining full passive ROM for flexion. Do not begin passive extension stretching at this time. A restraining extension splint may be used and positioned in available range if tightness is noted.
6 weeks	• Begin passive extension exercises of wrist and digits. • Fit extension resting pan splint in maximum extension if extrinsic flexor tendon tightness is significant; frequently the patient may need only an extension gutter splint for night wear.
8 weeks	• Begin resistive exercises with sponges or a Nerf ball and progress to putty and a hand-helper. Allow use of the hand in light work activities but no lifting or heavy use of the hand. • Allow full use of the hand in all daily activities. • Use work simulator or strengthening program to improve hand strength.
10 to 12 weeks	

The greatest achievement in total motion is seen between 12 to 14 weeks after surgery. It is not uncommon to see the patient begin to plateau in ROM between 6 to 8 weeks.

In patients with associated digital nerve repair with some degree of tension at the nerve site, the patient should be fitted with a separate digital dorsal blocking splint in 30 degrees of PIP joint flexion. This splint is worn for 6 weeks and is progressively adjusted into increased extension during that time frame (see the section on digital nerve repair).

REHABILITATION PROTOCOL

Early Mobilization of Immediate (or Delayed Primary) Repair of Zones 4 and 5: Modified Duran Protocol*

Prerequisites:	compliant patient clean or healed wound repair within 14 days of injury

7 to 14 days	• Remove bulky compressive dressing and apply light compressive dressing. Use digital-level finger socks or Coban.
	• Fit DBS to wrist and digits for continual wear in the following position:
	    Wrist—30 degrees of palmar flexion.
	    MCP joints—50 degrees of flexion.
	    PIP and DIP joints—full extension.
	• Begin hourly passive ROM exercises in flexion and extension within restraints of DBS. (See Figs. 1-1, 1-2, and 1-3.)

3 weeks	• Begin active ROM exercises (including blocking) 10 to 15 minutes each hour;

exercises may be performed within restraints of DBS.

• FES or electrical muscle stimulation (EMS) may be initiated to improve tendon excursion within 2 days of initiation of active ROM.

• Begin scar massage, scar retraction, and scar remodeling techniques to remodel scar tissue and minimize subcutaneous adhesions.

4.5 weeks	• Begin active ROM exercises of wrist and digits outside of DBS. If nerve repair has been done at wrist level, ROM exercises are performed within the splint to alleviate additional stress at nerve repair site. (See the section on nerve repairs.) *Continued*

REHABILITATION PROTOCOL—cont'd

Early Mobilization of Immediate (or Delayed Primary) Repair of Zones 4 and 5: Modified Duran Protocol*

6 weeks	• Discontinue DBS. • Begin passive ROM exercises of wrist and digits. • A full-extension resting pan splint or a long dorsal outrigger with a lumbrical bar may be used if extrinsic flexor tightness is present. Generally, this type of splinting is necessary with this level of repair. • Do not allow lifting or heavy use of the hand. • May begin gentle strengthening with a Nerf ball or putty.
7 weeks	• May upgrade progressive strengthening to include use of a hand-helper.
10 to 12 weeks	• Allow full use of the injured hand.

Once active ROM exercise is begun at 3 weeks, it is important to emphasize blocking exercises along with the composite active ROM exercises. If the patient is having difficulty recapturing active flexion, it is important to monitor progress carefully and request frequent patient visits to maximize flexion. *The first 3 to 7 weeks after surgery are critical for restoring tendon excursion.*

REHABILITATION PROTOCOL

Immediate (or Delayed Primary) Repair of Injuries in Zone 1, 2, or 3: Modified Early Motion Program*

Prerequisites:	compliant, motivated patient good repair, wound healing	

1 to 3 days	• Remove bulky compressive dressing and apply light compressive dressing.
	• Use digital-level finger socks or Coban for edema at digital level.
	• Fit DBS to wrist and digits for continual wear in the following position:
	  Wrist—20 degrees of palmar flexion.
	  MCP joints—50 degrees of flexion.
	  DIP and PIP joints—full extension.
	• Begin hourly passive ROM exercises in flexion and extension within restraints of DBS. (Refer to modified Duran protocol on p. 4.)	

3 weeks	• Begin active ROM exercises in flexion and extension within restraints of DBS 4 to 6 times a day, in addition to modified Duran protocol. (See p. 4.)	
4.5 weeks	• Begin hourly active ROM exercises of wrist and digits outside splint. • Patient should wear DBS between exercise sessions and at night.	
5.5 weeks	• Begin blocking exercises of DIP and PIP joint, as outlined in modified Duran protocol. (See Figs. 1-1 and 1-2.)	

Continued

REHABILITATION PROTOCOL—cont'd

Immediate (or Delayed Primary) Repair of Injuries in Zone 1, 2, or 3: Modified Early Motion Program*

6 weeks	• Discontinue DBS.
	• Begin passive ROM exercises in extension of wrist and digits as needed.
	• Begin extension splinting if extrinsic flexor tendon tightness or PIP joint contracture is present.
8 weeks	• Begin progressive strengthening.
	• Do not allow lifting or heavy use of the hand.
10 to 12 weeks	• Allow full use of hand, including sports.

This protocol differs from the modified Duran protocol because the patient may begin active ROM exercises within the restraints of the DBS at 3 weeks instead of exercising out of the splint at 4.5 weeks.

REHABILITATION PROTOCOL

Noncompliant Patient With Injury in Zones 1 Through 5: Delayed Mobilization*

Indications: crush injury
younger than 11 years of age
poor compliance and/or intelligence
soft tissue loss, wound management problems

3 weeks
- Remove bulky dressing and apply light compressive dressing.
- Fit DBS to wrist and digits for continual wear in the following position:
  Wrist—30 degrees of palmar flexion
  MCP joints—50 degrees of flexion
  PIP and DIP joints—full extension
- Begin hourly active and passive ROM exercises within restraints of DBS; blocking exercises of PIP and DIP joints may be included.

- Active ROM is begun earlier than in other protocols because of longer (3 weeks) immobilization in DBS.

4.5 weeks
- Begin active ROM exercises of digits and wrist outside of DBS; continue passive ROM exercises within restraints of splint.
- May use FES or EMS to improve tendon excursion.
- If an associated nerve repair is under any degree of tension, continue exercises within DBS that are appropriate for the level of nerve repair.

Continued

REHABILITATION PROTOCOL—cont'd

Noncompliant Patient With Injury in Zones 1 Through 5: Delayed Mobilization*

6 weeks	• Discontinue DBS. • Begin passive ROM exercises in extension of wrist and digits. • May use extension resting pan splint for extrinsic flexor tendon tightness or joint stiffness. • Do not allow lifting or heavy use of hand.
8 weeks	• Begin progressive strengthening with putty and hand-helper.
10 to 12 weeks	• Allow full use of hand.

This delayed mobilization program for digital-level to forearm-level flexor tendon repairs is reserved primarily for significant crush injuries, which may include severe edema or wound problems. This program is best used for patients whose primary repair may be somewhat "ragged" because of the crushing or bursting nature of the wound. It also is indicated for young children who cannot comply with an early motion protocol, such as the modified Duran program. *It is not indicated for patients who have a simple primary repair.*

REHABILITATION PROTOCOL

Repair of Flexor Pollicis Longus (FPL) of Thumb: Early Mobilization*

Prerequisites:	compliant patient clean or healed wound
1 to 3 days	• Remove bulky compressive dressing and apply light compressive dressing; use finger socks or coban on thumb for edema control. • Fit DBS to wrist and thumb for continual wear in the following position: Wrist—20 degrees of palmar flexion Thumb MCP and interphalangeal (IP) joints—15 degrees of flexion at each joint Thumb carpometacarpal (CMC) joint—palmar abduction
	■ *It is important to ensure that the thumb IP joint is in 15 degrees of flexion and is not extended. When the IP joint is left in a neutral position, restoration of IP flexion can be difficult.*
	• Begin hourly controlled passive mobilization program within restraints of DBS: 8 repetitions passive flexion and extension of MCP joint (Fig. 1-6).
	8 repetitions passive flexion and extension of IP joint (Fig. 1-7). 8 repetitions passive flexion and extension in composite manner of MCP and IP joints (Fig. 1-8).
4.5 weeks	• Remove DBS each hour to allow performance of the following exercises: 10 repetitions active flexion and extension of wrist (Fig. 1-9). 10 repetitions active flexion and extension of thumb (Fig. 1-10). • Continue passive ROM exercises. • Patient should wear DBS between exercise sessions and at night.
5 weeks	• May use FES or EMS within restraints of DBS to improve tendon excursion. *Continued*

REHABILITATION PROTOCOL—cont'd

Repair of Flexor Pollicis Longus (FPL) of Thumb: Early Mobilization*

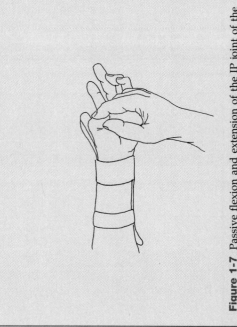

Figure 1-6 Passive flexion and extension of the MCP joint of the thumb.*

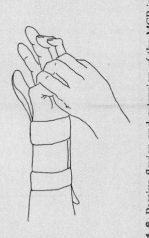

Figure 1-7 Passive flexion and extension of the IP joint of the thumb.*

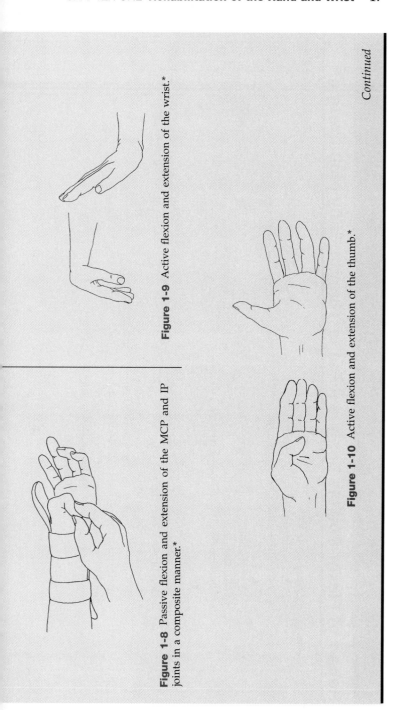

Figure 1-8 Passive flexion and extension of the MCP and IP joints in a composite manner.*

Figure 1-9 Active flexion and extension of the wrist.*

Figure 1-10 Active flexion and extension of the thumb.*

Continued

REHABILITATION PROTOCOL—cont'd

Repair of Flexor Pollicis Longus (FPL) of Thumb: Early Mobilization*

5.5 weeks
- Discontinue DBS.
- Begin hourly active ROM exercises:
  12 repetitions blocking of thumb IP joint (Fig. 1-11).
  12 repetitions composite active flexion and extension of thumb.
- Continue passive ROM exercises as necessary.

6 weeks
- Begin passive ROM exercises in extension of wrist and thumb.
- If needed for extrinsic flexor tendon tightness in the FPL, a wrist and thumb static splint can be used to hold the wrist and thumb in extension. Often, a simple extension gutter splint in full extension can be used for night wear.

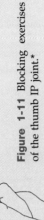

Figure 1-11 Blocking exercises of the thumb IP joint.*

8 weeks	• Begin progressive strengthening with a Nerf ball and progress to a hand-helper. • Do not allow lifting or heavy use of hand.
10 to 12 weeks	• Allow full use of the hand for most activities, including sports. • ROM generally begins to plateau at approximately 7 to 8 weeks after surgery.

• If an associated digital nerve repair is under tension, position the thumb in 30 degrees of flexion at the MCP and IP joints.
• If passive flexion is limited, taping or dynamic flexion splinting may be used.
• Scar management, including scar retraction, scar massage, and the use of Otoform or Elastomer, may be used at 2 weeks after surgery.

REHABILITATION PROTOCOL

Repair of Flexor Pollicis Longus (FPL) of Thumb: Delayed Mobilization*

Indications: crush injury

patient younger than 7 years of age poor compliance and/or intelligence soft tissue loss, wound management problems

The delayed mobilization program for FPL repairs is best reserved for patients with crush injuries, soft tissue loss, wound management problems, and patients in whom end-to-end repair was difficult.

3 weeks

- Remove bulky compressive dressing and apply light compressive dressing; use finger sock or Coban as needed for edema control.
- Fit DBS to wrist and thumb for continual wear in the following position:
  Wrist—30 degrees of palmar flexion

Thumb CMC joint—palmar abduction
Thumb MCP and IP joints—15 degrees of flexion at each joint

- Begin hourly active and passive ROM exercises within restraints of DBS, including blocking exercises.
- If passive flexion of thumb is limited, tapping or dynamic flexion splinting may be used.
- Begin scar massage and scar management techniques.

4.5 weeks

- Begin hourly active ROM exercises of wrist and thumb outside splint.
- May use FES or EMS to improve tendon excursion of FPL.

Time	Intervention
6 weeks	• Discontinue DBS. • Begin passive ROM exercises in extension of wrist and thumb. • If extrinsic flexor tendon tightness of FPL is present, a wrist and thumb static splint may be used as needed; the patient should wear the splint between exercise sessions and at night. • Do not allow lifting or heavy use of the hand.
8 weeks	• Begin progressive strengthening with a Nerf ball or putty.
10 to 12 weeks	• Allow full use of hand for most activities. • If associated digital nerve repair is under tension, position thumb MCP and IP joints in 30 degrees of flexion to minimize tension at repair site. • Composite active flexion of the thumb tends to reach a plateau between 9 and 10 weeks after surgery.

REHABILITATION PROTOCOL

Two-Stage Reconstruction for Delayed Tendon Repair*

Stage 1 (Hunter rod)

BEFORE SURGERY

- Maximize passive ROM of digit with manual passive exercises, digital level taping, or dynamic splinting.
- Use scar management techniques to improve suppleness of soft tissues, including scar massage, scar retraction, and use of Otoform or Elastomer silicone molds.
- Begin strengthening exercises of future donor tendon to improve postoperative strength after stage 2 procedure.
- If needed for protection or assistance with ROM, use buddy taping of the involved digit.

AFTER SURGERY

5 to 7 days
- Remove bulky dressing and apply light compressive dressing; use digital-level finger socks or coban.

- Begin active and passive ROM exercises of hand for approximately 10 minutes, 6 times each day.
- Fit an extension gutter splint that holds the digit in full extension to wear between exercise sessions and at night.
- If pulleys have been reconstructed during stage 1, use taping for about 8 weeks during the postoperative phase.

3 to 6 weeks
- Gradually wean patient from extension gutter splint; continue buddy taping for protection.

■ *The major goal during stage 1 is to maintain passive ROM and obtain supple soft tissues before tendon grafting.*

Stage 2 (free tendon graft)
AFTER SURGERY

- Follow instructions for early motion program for zones 1 through 3 (modified Duran protocol) on p. 4 or the delayed mobilization program for zones 1 through 5 on p. 13.

- For most patients, the modified Duran program is preferable to the delayed mobilization program because it encourages greater excursion of the graft and helps maintain passive ROM through the early mobilization exercises.

- Do not use FES before 5 to 5.5 weeks after surgery because of the initial avascularity of the tendon graft. Also consider the reasons for failure of the primary repair.

Extensor Tendon Injuries

REHABILITATION RATIONALE AND BASIC PRINCIPLES

Anatomy

Extensor mechanism injuries are conveniently grouped into eight anatomic zones according to Kleinert and Verdan (Table 1-1; see Figs. 1-12, 1-13, and 1-14).

Treatment: Zones 1 and 2 Extensor Tendon Injuries

Closed mallet injuries in adults are managed with 6 weeks of splinting with a mallet-finger splint that holds the DIP joint in extension. When external splinting is not possible or when a mallet deformity results from an acute open injury, pinning for 6 weeks with a 0.045 Kirschner wire may be preferred. The wire is removed at 6 weeks and the remainder of the closed extensor program is followed.

Bony mallet deformities may be managed closed, unless the fragment is 50% or more of the articular surface. This may result in joint subluxation, and pin fixation and open reduction may be required. In any event, 6 weeks of immobilization precedes initiation of DIP exercises with interval splinting.

Mallet injuries that do not respond to a splinting program and those of 3 to 6 months duration are classified as *chronic*. Further splinting may be attempted, with full extension splinting for 8 weeks initially, or, if the deformity is unacceptable, surgical correction may be indicated. Motion-preserving procedures are re-

TABLE 1-1 **Zones of Injury**

| | Extensor | |
Zone	Finger	Thumb
1	DIP joint	IP joint
2	Middle phalanx	Proximal phalanx
3	Apex PIP joint	MCP joint
4	Proximal phalanx	Metacarpal
5	Apex MCP joint	
6	Dorsal hand	
7	Dorsal retinaculum	Dorsal retinaculum
8	Distal forearm	Distal forearm

From Kleinert HE, Verdan C: Report of the Committee on Tendon Injuries, *J Hand Surg* 8:794, 1983.

served for nonarthritic DIP joints with a minimum passive ROM of 50 degrees. Fixed deformities and painful degenerative joints are best managed by arthrodesis.

Rehabilitation
Extensor tendon treatment protocol selection depends on the mechanism of injury and the time elapsed since the injury. The following protocols apply to isolated zonal extensor tendon disruptions.

Clearly, modifications of these programs will be dictated by other concomitant injuries.

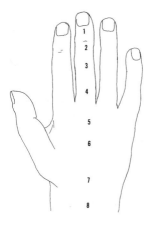

Figure 1-12 Zones of the extensor tendons.

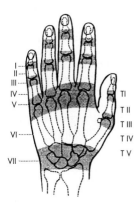

Figure 1-13 Extensor tendon zones. (From Kleinert HE, Schepel S, Gill T: Flexor tendon injuries, *Surg Clin North Am* 61:267, 1981.)

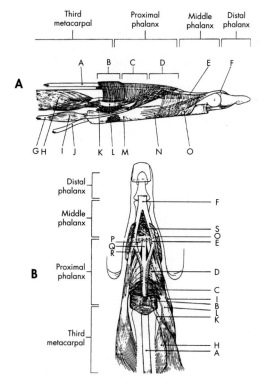

Figure 1-14 Diagrammatic representation of dorsal apparatus of finger. **A,** Radial side of left middle finger. **B,** Dorsum of left middle finger. *A,* Extensor digitorum communis tendon; *B,* sagittal bands; *C,* transverse fibers of intrinsic muscle apparatus; *D,* oblique fibers of intrinsic apparatus; *E,* conjoined lateral band; *F,* terminal tendon; *G,* flexor digitorum profundus tendon; *H,* second dorsal interosseous muscle; *I,* lumbrical muscle; *J,* flexor digitorum superficialis tendon; *K,* medial tendon of superficial belly of interosseous; *L,* lateral tendon of deep belly of interosseous; *M,* flexor pulley mechanism; *N,* oblique retinacular ligament; *O,* transverse retinacular ligament; *P,* medial band of oblique fibers of intrinsic expansion; *Q,* central slip; *R,* lateral slips; *S,* triangular ligament. (From Smith RJ: Balance and kinetics of the fingers under normal and pathological conditions, *Clin Orthop* 104:95, 1974.)

REHABILITATION PROTOCOL

Acute Extensor Tendon Injuries in Zones 1 and 2

0 to 6 weeks	• Treat closed mallet injuries of adults with a mallet finger splint with the DIP joint in 0 to 15 degrees of of hyperextension. • Apply the mallet splint volar or dorsal to allow sensory input to the palmar surface of the finger. • Permit splint removal for hygienic purposes while the ipsilateral thumb maintains the splinted posture of the DIP joint. • Encourage full MCP and PIP joint motion during splinting.
6 to 9 weeks	• Begin weaning from the splint if no extensor lag is present after splint removal. Begin active DIP flexion with interval splinting between hourly exercises. Continue night splinting until the eighth week. • Should a DIP joint extensor lag exceed 10 degrees after the initial 6-week splinting period, reinstitute night splinting for 2 more weeks or until a satisfactory result is obtained.

EXTENSOR TENDON INJURIES IN ZONES 4, 5, AND 6

Normal function usually is possible after unilateral injuries to the dorsal apparatus, and splinting and immobilization are not recommended. Complete disruptions of the dorsal expansion or central slip lacerations are repaired.

Zone 5 extensor tendon subluxations rarely respond to a splinting program. The affected MCP joint may be splinted in full extension and radial deviation for 4 weeks with the understanding that surgical intervention probably will be required. Painful popping and swelling, in addition to a problematic extensor lag with radial deviation of the involved digit, usually require prompt reconstruction. Please refer to *Clinical Orthopaedic Rehabilitation* textbook for rehabilitation protocols covering zones 7 and 8 and the extensor subluxations of zone 5.

EPL Repairs

Repairs performed 3 weeks or longer after the injury may weaken the extensor pollicis longus (EPL) muscle sufficiently for electrical stimulation to become necessary for tendon glide. The EPL is selectively strengthened by thumb retropulsion exercises performed against resistance with the palm held on a flat surface.

REHABILITATION PROTOCOL

Extensor Tendon Injury in Zone 4, 5, or 6, After Surgical Repair

0 to 2 weeks	• Allow active and passive PIP exercises; keep the MCP joint in full extension and the wrist in 40 degrees of extension.	4 to 6 weeks	• Begin MCP and wrist joint active flexion exercises with interval and night splinting with the wrist in neutral position.
			• Over the next 2 weeks, begin active-assisted and gentle passive flexion exercises.
2 weeks	• Remove the sutures and fit the patient with a removable splint	6 weeks	• Discontinue splinting unless an extensor lag develops at the MCP joint.
	• Keep the MCP joints in full extension and the wrist in neutral position.		• Use passive wrist flexion exercises as necessary.
	• Continue PIP exercises and remove the splint for scar massage and hygienic purposes only.		

REHABILITATION PROTOCOL

Extensor Pollicis Longus Laceration

After repair of thumb extensor tendon lacerations, regardless of the zone of injury, apply a thumb spica splint with the wrist in 30 degrees of extension and the thumb in 40 degrees of radial abduction with full retroposition.

0 to 2 weeks

- Allow activity as comfortable in the postoperative splint.
- Edema control measures include elevation and motion exercises to uninvolved digits.

2 to 4 weeks

- At 2 weeks after repair, remove the splint and sutures. Refit a thumb spica splint with the wrist and thumb positioned to minimize tension at the repair site as before.
- Fit a removable splint for reliable patients and permit scar massage.
- The vocational interests of some patients are best suited with a thumb spica cast. Continue edema control measures.

4 to 6 weeks

- Fit a removable thumb spica splint for night use and interval daily splinting between exercises.
- During the next 2 weeks, the splint is removed for hourly wrist and thumb exercises. Between weeks 4 and 5 the patient should perform the thumb IP, MCP, and CMC flexion and extension exercises with the wrist held in extension.
- Alternately, wrist flexion and extension motion is regained with the thumb extension.
- After the fifth week, perform composite wrist and thumb exercises concomitantly.

6 weeks

- Discontinue the splinting program unless extensor lags develop.
- Treat an extensor lag at the IP joint of more than 10 degrees with intermittent IP extension splinting in addition to nightly thumb spica splinting.

6 weeks— cont'd

- Problematic MCP and CMC extension lags require intermittent thumb spica splinting during the day and night for an additional 2 weeks or until acceptable results are obtained.

- It may be necessary to continue edema control measures to 8 weeks or longer after surgery.
- May use taping to gain full composite thumb flexion.
- May use electrical stimulation for lack of extensor pull through.

DEQUERVAIN'S TENOSYNOVITIS

Stenosing tenosynovitis of the abductor pollicis longus (APL) and extensor pollicis brevis (EPB) tendons usually causes discomfort localized to the region of the radial styloid (Fig. 1-15, *A*). Tenderness and swelling over the first dorsal compartment are usually accompanied by a positive Finkelstein's test (Fig. 1-15, *B*); however, resisted thumb MCP extension may be the only sign in more subtle cases.

Conservative management

Thumb spica splint—immobilize the first dorsal compartment tendons with the use of a commercially available splint or, depending on the patient's comfort, a custom-molded orthoplast device. The splint maintains the wrist in 15 to 20 degrees of extension and the thumb in 30 degrees of radial and palmar abduction. The IP joint is left free, and motion at this joint is encouraged. The patient wears the splint during the day for the first 2 weeks and at night until the next office visit, generally at 6 to 8 weeks. Splinting may continue longer, depending on the response to this form of treatment. Discontinue the splint during the day if symptoms permit and if daily activities are gradually resumed. Tailor workplace advancement accordingly.

Corticosteroid injection—offer a steroid injection to patients with moderate to marked pain or with symptoms lasting more than 3 weeks. The injection should distend individually the APL and

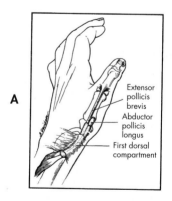

Figure 1-15 A, the anatomic arrangement of the first dorsal extensor compartment. The tunnel contains the extensor pollicis brevis tendon and one or more slips of the abductor pollicis longus tendon.

EPB sheaths. Postinjection discomfort is variable, and a 2- to 3-day supply of mild analgesic is recommended.

Antiinflammatory agent—a systemic nonsteroidal antiinflammatory agent is commonly prescribed for the initial 6 to 8 weeks of treatment.

Activity modification—restrict thumb use so that the first dorsal compartment tendons are at relative rest. Avoid activities that require prolonged thumb IP joint flexion, pinch, or repetitive motions.

Therapeutic modalities—edema control may be attempted through distal-to-proximal thumb coban wrapping, retrograde lotion or ice massage over the radial styloid, and phonophoresis with 10% hydrocortisone. Perform gentle active and passive thumb and wrist motion 5 minutes hourly to prevent joint contracture and tendon adhesions.

Often symptoms are temporarily relieved and the patient elects to repeat the management outlined above. Unsatisfactory symptom reduction or symptom persistence requires surgical decompression.

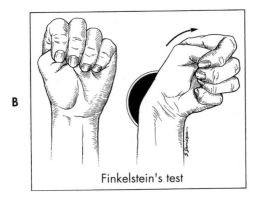

B

Finkelstein's test

Figure 1-15—cont'd B, Finkelstein's test. Flexion and ulnar deviation of the wrist with the fingers flexed over the thumb. Pain over the first compartment strongly suggests deQuervain's stenosing tenosynovitis. (From Strickland JW, Idler RS, Creighton JC: Hand clinic: DeQuervain's stenosing tenosynovitis, *Indiana Med* 83(5):340, 1990.)

Decompression for deQuervain's Tenosynovitis

0 to 2 days

- Leave the IP joint free and encourage motion as allowed by the soft compressive surgical dressing.
- 2 days after surgery, remove the dressing.
- Begin gentle active motion of the wrist and thumb.

2 to 14 days

- The presurgical splint is worn for comfort and motion exercises are continued.
- At the tenth to fourteenth day, remove the sutures.

- Commonly, patients complain of some hypersensitivity and of numbness at and distal to the incision site. Desensitization may be necessary. Digital massage of the area is usually sufficient, since the disturbance nearly always resolves.

2 to 6 weeks

- Advance the strengthening program and continue desensitization as necessary.
- Anticipate the patient's release to unrestricted activity no earlier than about 6 weeks after surgery.

Nerve Compression Syndromes

CARPAL TUNNEL SYNDROME

Treatment

Regardless of the severity of this compression neuropathy, the first line of managment is to decrease the inciting and aggravating factors. Patients should avoid repetitive gripping and squeezing, and palmar impaction forces should be minimized. Patients should be educated about ergonomics and changes that may be required at work.

For *mild to moderate symptoms,* a forearm-based wrist splint, with the wrist in neutral position, is worn 24 hours a day for 2 weeks or until symptoms subside. Night splinting is continued for 6 weeks or longer. Although splinting appears to be the most effective treatment for nocturnal paresthesias, nonsteroidal antiinflammatory medications may be prescribed in addition to vitamin B_6. Activity modifications also may be helpful.

Patients with *severe symptoms* may benefit from steroid injection into the carpal tunnel; injections can be repeated several times, depending on the patient's response. Conservative treatment usually is not beneficial for patients with symptoms of more than 6 months duration, with objective neurologic loss, with recurrent carpal tunnel syndrome, or with symptoms that followed blunt trauma to the wrist.

CUBITAL TUNNEL SYNDROME

Few patients with cubital tunnel syndrome respond to nonsurgical measures, but modification of workplace activities, including a decrease in forceful grip use of the hand and prolonged elbow flexion, may be beneficial. Long-arm night splints with the elbow in 40 degrees of flexion, antiinflammatory medication, and vitamin B_6 are prescribed. Elbow pads to decrease impaction on the cubital tunnel also are worthwhile, especially if the cubital tunnel syndrome is accompanied by medial epicondylitis. Nonsurgical management for this disorder may be used as long as the patient desires, but 3 to 6 months seems reasonable.

Postsurgical therapy for cubital tunnel syndrome depends on the surgical technique used.

REHABILITATION PROTOCOL

Carpal Tunnel Syndrome: Open Release

0 to 7 days	• Encourage wrist extension and flexion exercises and full finger flexion and extension exercises immediately after surgery in the postsurgical dressing.
7 days	• Remove the dressing. Prohibit the patient from submerging the hand in liquids but permit showering. Discontinue the wrist splint if the patient is comfortable.
7 to 14 days	• Permit the patient to use the hand in activities of daily living as pain allows.
2 weeks	• Remove the sutures and begin ROM and gradual strengthening exercises. Achieve initial scar remodeling by using Elastomer or silicon gel-sheet scar pad at night and deep scar massage. If scar tenderness is intense, use desensitization techniques such as applying various textures to the area using light pressure and progressing to deep pressure. Textures include cotton, velour, wool, and Velcro.
	• Control pain and edema with the use of Isotoner gloves or electrical stimulation.
2 to 4 weeks	• Advance the patient to more rigorous activities; allow the patient to return to work if pain permits. The patient can use a padded glove for tasks that require pressure to be applied over the tender palmar scars. Begin pinch/grip strengthening with Baltimore Therapeutic Equipment work-simulator activities.

REHABILITATION PROTOCOL

Carpal Tunnel Syndrome: Endoscopic Release

0 to 1 day	• Encourage wrist extension and flexion exercises in the soft postsurgical dressing.
2 days	• Remove the dressing. Protect wounds from immersion in liquids. Encourage activities as palmar tenderness allows.
2 weeks	• Remove the sutures and advance activities to pain tolerance. Pillar tenderness (pain over the divided radial and ulnar portions of the transverse carpal ligament) may continue as a source of considerable discomfort and delay return to heavy work activities for 6 to 10 weeks after surgery.

REHABILITATION PROTOCOL

Cubital Tunnel Syndrome: In Situ Decompression

0 to 7 days	• Fit the patient with a long-arm splint with the elbow at 90 degrees of flexion and the forearm in neutral position. • Emphasize shoulder and digital motion.
7 days	• Remove the splint and apply a light compressive dressing to the elbow. Begin elbow, forearm, and wrist active and active-assisted exercises. • Control edema with high-voltage galvanic stimulator (HVGS). • Instruct the patient to avoid repetitive activities.
2 weeks	• Remove the sutures and begin an active ROM program. Emphasize full elbow extension, flexion, and forearm pronation and supination. Continue edema control, scar management, and desensitization as necessary.
4 weeks	• Begin resistive strengthening exercises for forearm pronation and supination, wrist curls, and grip/pinch exercises.
6 weeks	• Allow full activity.

REHABILITATION PROTOCOL

Medial Epicondylectomy and Anterior Transposition Procedure

0 to 2 weeks	• Fit the patient with a long-arm splint that keeps the elbow in 90 degrees of flexion, the forearm in 40 degrees pronation, and the wrist in 40 degrees of flexion. Encourage thumb and finger ROM. • Remove the sutures at 2 weeks.
2 to 4 weeks	• Fashion a removable long-arm splint to keep the elbow at 90 degrees of flexion and the forearm and wrist in neutral. The splint is removed hourly for 10-minute sessions of gentle active elbow, forearm, and wrist motion. Begin edema control with compression sleeve (tubi-grip), retrograde massage, and HVGS. • Begin scar management.
4 weeks	• Discontinue the splint. Advance from active and active-assisted elbow exercises to passive to regain full motion. Full concomitant forearm and wrist motion should be present at 4 weeks.
5 weeks	• Begin strengthening exercises: wrist curls and forearm rotation Velcro board activities for wrist flexion, extension, pronation/supination, and pinch; hand-helper for grip.
6 weeks	• Allow activity as comfort permits. Begin gradual repetitive activities.
8 weeks	• Allow full unrestricted activity.

Nerve Injuries

Nerve injuries are most commonly caused by direct trauma, laceration, traction or stretching, entrapment, or compression. Obtaining optimal hand function after nerve injury depends on preservation of passive range of motion of the hand and prevention of secondary damage from attenuation or stretching of involved structures due to poor positioning or substitution patterns. Combined with the appropriate exercise regimens, splinting techniques can be effective for attaining these goals.

Median nerve lesions result in a loss of coordination, decreased strength, and a decrease in or loss of sensory input from the thumb, index, long, and ring fingers. Distal lesions primarily impair opposition and adduction, and splinting is aimed primarily at preventing first web contracture and maintaining passive motion of the thumb CMC joint.

Ulnar nerve lesions compromise coordination, pinch and grip strength, and thumb stability and frequently cause "clawing" of the ring and small fingers. Splinting is aimed at prevention of this clawing, while allowing full digital flexion and IP extension.

Radial nerve lesions result in loss of active extension of the wrist, thumb and fingers, weakness of thumb abduction, decreased grip strength, and diminished coordination. The emphasis of splinting is on providing wrist stability and maintaining thumb position.

SPLINTING FOR NERVE PALSIES*

Median nerve
Splint recommendation: web spacer

Purpose	• The web spacer splint maintains the width of the first web space, preventing a first web contracture.
	• This is necessary because of the paralysis of the thenar musculature.
Warning/ Precautions	• When fabricating the splint, avoid hyperextension of the thumb MCP joint or stress to the ulnar collateral ligament (UCL) of the MCP joint.
Wearing Time	• Night only.
	• If any first web space contracture is noted, periodic daywear is added.

Ulnar nerve

Splint recommendation: single Wynn-Parry splint or static MCP extension block.

Purpose	• These splints are used to prevent clawing of the ring and small fingers, yet allow full digital flexion and IP extension.
	• The splint is required because of paralysis of the ulnar innervated intrinsics.
Warning/ Precautions	• Monitor carefully to prevent pressure sores in patients who do not have sensory return.
Wearing Time	• Continuous wear until the MCP volar plates tighten so that hyperextension is no longer present, the intrinsics return, or tendon transfers are performed to replace the function of the intrinsics.

Radial nerve

Splint recommendation: wrist immobilization splint or possibly a long dorsal outrigger.

Purpose	• Positioning the wrist in approximately 15 to 20 degrees of dorsiflexion allows improved functional use of the hand and prevents wrist drop.
	• Incorporation of the outrigger component of the splint allows assistance with extension at the MCP level of the digits.
Wearing Time	• The patient wears the splint until there is return of the radial nerve innervated muscles or tendon transfers are performed to improve wrist and/or finger extension.

DIGITAL NERVE REPAIR

Most lacerations of digital nerves should be repaired as soon as possible (within 5 to 7 days of injury) if the wound is clean and sharp. The condition of the patient, the presence of other injuries that may take precedence over nerve repair, skin conditions such as extensive soft-tissue loss, wound contamination, and the availability of personnel and equipment also must be considered in the timing of digital nerve repair.

REHABILITATION PROTOCOL

Repair of Digital Nerve*

2 weeks	• Remove bulky dressing and initiate edema control with coban or finger socks. • Fit DBS in 30 degrees of flexion at the PIP joint for continual wear, assuming the repair is near the PIP level or slightly distal to this point. The DBS may be fitted in more flexion at the MCP or PIP level if the digital nerve repair is under more tension. **Note:** If nerve repair is near the MCP joint, the DBS should include the MCP joint only, with approximately 30 degrees of flexion of the MCP joint. • Begin active and passive ROM exercises 6 times a day within the restraints of the dorsal blocking gutter. • Begin scar massage with lotion and/or the use of Otoform or Elastomer within 24 hours after suture removal.
3 to 6 weeks	• Adjust the dorsal blocking gutter splint into extension 10 degrees each week until neutral is reached at 6 weeks.
6 weeks	• Discontinue DBS. • Initiate passive extension at the MCP joint. • May begin extension splinting if passive extension is limited, but generally patients regain extension and extension splints are not necessary. • Begin progressive strengthening.
8 to 10 weeks	• Begin sensory reeducation when some sign of sensory return (protective sensation) is present.

REHABILITATION PROTOCOL

Excision of Wrist Ganglion Cyst

2 weeks	• Remove the short-arm splint and sutures. Initiate active and active-assisted wrist extension and flexion. Continue interval splint wear during the day between exercises and at night.
2 to 4 weeks	• Advance ROM exercises to resistive and gradual strengthening exercises. • Discontinue the splint at 4 weeks.
4 to 6 weeks	• Allow normal activities to tolerance.
6 weeks	• Allow full activity.

The time it takes to achieve full wrist extension and flexion depends on the the patient. Return of motion, however, is quite predictable, and only rarely is formal therapy necessary after 4 to 6 weeks.

RHEUMATOID ARTHRITIS

The radioulnar joint is a frequent site of proliferative synovitis in patients with rheumatoid arthritis. Progressive synovitis of the distal radioulnar joint results in dorsal subluxation and sometimes dislocation of the ulnar head. Synovectomy of the distal radioulnar joint often is combined with resection of the ulnar head (Darrach procedure) for the treatment of these problems.

REHABILITATION PROTOCOL

Darrach Resection of the Distal Ulna*

■ If the Darrach procedure is performed in conjunction with multiple procedures for rheumatoid arthritis, active ROM exercises may begin 3 to 5 days after surgery at the discretion of the physician. If the Darrach surgical area is painful, exercises may need to be minimized in the initial 2 to 3 weeks.

0 to 3 weeks

- Apply a bulky compressive splint with the forearm supinated and the elbow flexed 90 degrees.
- At 2 weeks, replace the bulky dressing with a long-arm splint.

3 weeks

- Fit a wrist immobilization splint with 15 degrees of dorsiflexion to wear between exercise sessions and at night (some authors prefer to use a long-arm splint until 6 weeks after surgery).
- Begin hourly active and passive ROM exercises to the wrist and forearm. **Be sure to perform passive exercises proximal to the wrist and not distally by turning the hand.**
- Discomfort along the distal ulna when attempting forearm rotation is typical for the first 6 weeks.
- Patients with dorsal subluxation of the distal ulna may derive comfort from a distal ulnar strap applied 2 inches proximally to the distal ulna to help hold the ulna in an anatomic position.

6 weeks

- Discontinue wrist immobilization splint if the patient is experiencing no pain.
- Initiate gentle strengthening exercises.

Replantation

Replantation of amputated parts and revascularization for salvaging mangled extremities require intense commitment from both the patient and the surgeon. Emotional and financial investments are enormous, and successful replantation and revascularization require long postsurgical rehabilitation programs that are frequently interrupted and prolonged by multiple reconstructive surgical procedures.

▪ *Proper candidate selection is critical to the success of replantation and revascularization of amputated parts.*

CONTRAINDICATIONS

Absolute contraindications for replantation and revascularization include multiple-trauma victims with significant associated injuries in whom treatment of other organ systems takes precedence over extremity salvage. Digits have been refrigerated and replanted up to 3 days after injury. Extensive injury to the affected limb, chronic illness, previously nonfunctioning parts, and psychiatric illness also prohibit salvage procedures.

Relative contraindications include avulsion injuries, lengthy ischemia time, and patients older than 50 years. Major limbs are defined as those with significant skeletal muscle content. These may be salvaged if appropriately cooled 12 hours after the injury; up to 6 hours of warm ischemia time can be tolerated. Only under unusual circumstances should single digits be replanted, especially those proximal to the flexor digitorum superficialis insertion.

INDICATIONS

The ideal candidate for replantation is a young patient with a narrow zone of injury. Power saws and punch presses often result in replantable parts. Indications for replantation include any upper or lower extremity in a child, as well as thumbs, multiple digits, hands, and wrist-level and some more proximal-level amputations in adults.

POSTSURGICAL CONSIDERATIONS

Postsurgical care typically begins in the operating room, where brachial plexus blocks are given before the patient leaves. A bulky, noncompressive dressing reinforced with plaster splints is applied in the operating room and usually is kept in place for 3 weeks. When the likelihood of thrombosis is increased, such as in wide zone injuries, heparin may be used. Postsurgical orders include keeping the patient NPO for 12 to 24 hours after surgery, because vascular compromise may necessitate emergency surgical intervention. The replanted part is kept warm either with a thermal blanket or by elevating the room temperature to 78° to 80° F. Caffeine-containing products, such as coffee, tea, cola, and chocolate, are prohibited, as is smoking and the use of tobacco products by both the patient and visitors. Ice and iced drinks are not allowed, and visitation is limited to one to two visitors at a time to try to prevent emotional disturbance. The patient is restricted to bed rest for approximately 3 days, and the replanted part is kept at or slightly above heart level.

REHABILITATION PROTOCOL

Replantation and Revascularization in Adults

1 day

- Appropriate and liberal use of analgesics is recommended, although postoperative discomfort usually is minimal with replantations. Revascularization procedures typically require more postoperative pain management, especially when neural connections remain.

- Low-molecular-weight dextran 40 in 500 cc of D_5-W is given over 6 to 24 hours. In patients with pulmonary problems, continuous intravenous infusion at a lower rate is recommended.

- Aspirin (325 mg, 1 by mouth 2 times a day).

- Thorazine (25 mg by mouth 3 times a day).

- Antibiotics—cefazolin or a similar antibiotic is used for 3 to 5 days.

- Administer low-molecular-weight dextran 40 and 500 cc of D_5-W at a rate of 10 ml/kg/day for 3 days to the pediatric patient.

- Automated monitors with alarms provide continuous feedback, although hourly visual inspection for the first 12 hours provides important information, including color, capillary refill, turgor, and bleeding of the replanted part.

Management of Early Complications

- 5 to 10 days of hospitalization are necessary after replantation. After that time, replantation failure from vascular compromise occurs infrequently. Arterial insufficiency from thrombosis or vasoconstriction usually requires immediate return to the operating room. Give a plexus block, explore the arterial anastomosis, excise the damaged segment, and perform vein

Management of Early Complications—cont'd

grafting if necessary. Administer heparin in salvage procedures of this sort and attempt to keep the partial thromboplastin time 1.5 to 2.0 times normal.

- Venous congestion indicates either insufficient venous outflow or venous thrombosis. At the first sign of venous congestion, loosen all postoperative dressings to eliminate external constriction. Digital replantations with venous congestion may benefit from a longitudinal laceration through the digital pulp or removal of the nail plate. Heparinized-saline drops applied to the nail bed and pulp may promote venous drainage. If the venous outflow from the nail bed or drainage site is inadequate but present, leech therapy may be indicated. Apply a medical leech to the finger or area of congestion with the remaining sites shielded by plastic sheathing. A leech cage may be fashioned from the plastic bag in which intravenous bags are stored. Tape the open end of the plastic bag around the bulky postoperative dressing, introduce a leech through a vertical slit in the bag, then tape the vertical slit. Adequate oxygenization occurs through the porous surgical dressing. Leeches have a long-lasting anticoagulant and vasodilating effect in addition to withdrawing approximately 5 cc of blood. However, arterial inflow must be present for the leech to attach. If the leech does not attach, the digit may have arterial as well as venous insufficiency and further salvage requires immediate surgical exploration of the artery and venous anastomoses.

5 to 10 days

- The patient may be discharged from the hospital if the appearance of the replanted part is acceptable.
- Dietary and environmental restrictions remain the same, and the patient receives aspirin (325 mg) twice daily for an additional 2 weeks.

Continued

REHABILITATION·PROTOCOL—cont'd

Replantation and Revascularization in Adults

3 weeks	• Remove the dressing and assess the wound. Replanted digits usually are markedly edematous with granulating wounds. • Wound care management consists of hydrogen peroxide wound cleansing and silver nitrate cauterization of redundant granulation tissue. • Apply soft, nonadherent dressings and fit the wrist with a splint in slight wrist flexion and MCP joint flexion to about 50 to 60 degrees. • Begin passive wrist flexion and MCP joint flexion exercises, with emphasis on flexor tendon glide.	6 weeks	• Begin active and active-assisted ROM and flexion and extension with interval splinting. • Continue edema control measures.
		8 weeks	• Accelerate active and active-assisted flexion and extension exercises of all joints and use electrical stimulation if necessary. • Remove temporary bony fixation.
		4 months	• Perform soft tissue and bony reconstruction procedures. • PIP joint injuries are commonly treated by fusion. Active digital extension and flexion are often inhibited by tendon adhesions. • Motion is best achieved through a two-stage tenolysis program. Perform extensor tenolyses first, followed by a flexor tenolysis approximately 2 to 3 months after the initial procedure.

Arthroplasty

THUMB CARPOMETACARPAL JOINT ARTHROPLASTY

Treatment regimens with steroid injection, splinting, and nonsteroidal antiinflammatory agents should be exhausted before surgical intervention.

Total joint arthroplasty, implant arthroplasty, interposition arthroplasty, suspension arthroplasties, and CMC joint fusion have been used to alleviate pain and restore function in the diseased basilar joint of the thumb.

Silastic Trapezial Arthroplasty

The low-demand rheumatoid thumb is most suitable for silicone implant arthroplasty, because this implant has a 25% failure rate. More than 80% satisfactory results are reported, despite 56% scaphoid cysts and 74% intramedullary metacarpal radiolucency and/or cysts at long-term follow-up.

Interposition and Sling Suspension Arthroplasties

Trapezial excision techniques combined with soft tissue interposition or sling suspension arthroplasties have similar postsurgical protocols. Sling suspension arthroplasties are designed to prevent thumb osteoarticular column shortening and provide stability beyond that afforded by simple trapezial excision.

REHABILITATION PROTOCOL

Silastic Trapezial Arthroplasty

2 weeks	• Remove the well-padded volar surgical splint and surgical dressing, as well as the temporary Kirschner wire. • Apply a short-arm thumb spica cast.
6 weeks	• Remove the cast and begin controlled CMC, MCP, and IP active ROM exercises with interval protective thumb spica splinting.
9 weeks	• Discontinue the splinting.
3 to 6 months	• Allow the patient to resume normal activities of daily living.

REHABILITATION PROTOCOL

Interposition and Sling Suspension Arthroplasties

2 weeks	• Remove the surgical thumb spica splint and sutures. Apply a short-arm thumb spica cast for an additional 2 weeks.	8 weeks	• Encourage light to moderate activity. • The wrist and thumb static splint may be discontinued in the presence of a pain-free and stable joint.
4 weeks	• Begin active, active-assisted, and passive ROM exercises with interval splinting. • Ideally the splint or cast should include only CMC joint, leaving the MP or IP free for ROM.	3 months	• Allow normal activity.
			Discomfort frequently lasts for 6 months after surgery. The function and strength of the thumb will improve over a 6- to 12-month period.
6 weeks	• Begin gentle strengthening exercises.		

Fractures and Dislocations

Fractures and dislocations involving the hand are classified as stable or unstable injuries to determine the appropriate treatment. Stable fractures are those that should not displace if some degree of early digital motion is allowed. Unstable fractures are those that displace to an unacceptable degree if early digital motion is allowed. Although some unstable fractures can be converted to stable fractures with closed reduction, it is very difficult to predict which of these will maintain their stability throughout the early treatment phase. For this reason most unstable fractures should undergo closed reduction and percutaneous pinning or open reduction and internal fixation to allow for early protected digital motion and thus prevent stiffness.

METACARPAL AND PHALANGEAL FRACTURES

Nondisplaced metacarpal fractures are stable injuries and are treated with the application of an anterior-posterior splint in the *position of function:* the wrist in 30 to 60 degrees of extension, the MCP joints in 70 degrees of flexion, and the IP joints in 0 to 10 degrees of flexion. In this position, the important ligaments of the wrist and hand are maintained in maximum tension to prevent contractures.

Allowing early PIP and DIP joint motion is essential. Motion prevents adhesions between the tendons and the underlying fracture and controls edema. The dorsal fiberglass splint should extend from below the elbow to the fingertips of all of the involved digits and one adjacent digit. The anterior splint should extend from below the elbow to the distal aspect of the proximal phalanx (Fig. 1-16, *A*), allowing the patient to resume PIP and DIP active flexion and extension exercises immediately (Fig. 1-16, *B*).

Displaced transverse metacarpal fractures, after closed reduction, are treated similarly to nondisplaced fractures. Roentgenograms in the splint should be obtained at weekly intervals to be certain that acceptable skeletal alignment is maintained. Extension contractures of the MCP joints are common after metacarpal fractures and are caused by inadequate splinting in MCP flexion or excessive dorsal angulation of the metacarpal, resulting in intrinsic weakness and clawing. Extension contractures should be treated with aggressive, dynamic flexion splinting, such as a knuckle-bender splint.

Nondisplaced extraarticular phalangeal fractures are treated with similar anterior-posterior splints; however, the anterior splint must also extend out to the fingertips to support the fracture in the position of function. ROM exercises are begun at 3 weeks.

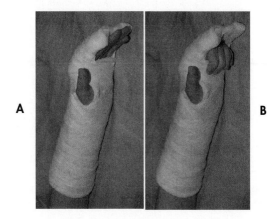

Figure 1-16 A and **B,** Anterior and posterior fiberglass splints typically used to treat metacarpal and proximal phalangeal fractures. PIP and DIP flexion and extension are allowed. The anterior splint should extend 2 cm distal to the level of the fracture.

Unstable metacarpal and phalangeal fractures require closed reduction and percutaneous pinning or open reduction and internal fixation. Stable fracture fixation is imperative to allow early ROM.

Comminuted phalangeal fractures, especially those that involve diaphyseal segments with thick cortices, may be slow to heal and may require fixation for up to 6 weeks (see protocol below).

0-4 weeks	• Before pin removal, begin active ROM exercises while the therapist supports the fracture site.
4-6 weeks	• Active and active-assisted intrinsic stretching exercises (i.e., simultaneous MCP extension and IP flexion) are recommended. • Prevent PIP joint flexion contractures by ensuring that the initial splint immobilizes the PIP joint in an almost neutral position. • When the fracture is considered solid on roentgenogram, a dynamic splinting program can be started. The LMB dynamic extension splint and the Capner splint are quite useful. They should be worn for 2-hour increments, 6 to 12 hours a day (Fig. 1-17), and alternated with dynamic flexion strapping (Fig. 1-18). • Therapy may be prolonged for up to 3 to 6 months after injury.

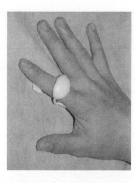

Figure 1-17 Dynamic PIP extension splint (LMB).

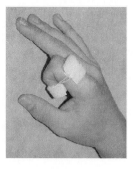

Figure 1-18 Flexion strap used to help regain PIP and DIP flexion.

Volar PIP joint dislocations are less common than dorsal dislocations and often are difficult to reduce by closed techniques because of entrapment of the lateral bands around the flare of the proximal phalangeal head. If not treated properly, these injuries may result in a boutonnière deformity (combined PIP flexion and DIP extension contracture). Usually the joint is stable after closed or open reduction; however, static PIP extension splinting is recommended for 6 weeks to allow healing of the central slip.

Avulsion fractures involving the dorsal margin of the middle phalanx occur at the insertion of the central slip. These fractures may be treated by closed technique; however, if the fragment is displaced more than 2 mm proximally with the finger splinted in extension, open reduction and internal fixation of the fragment are indicated.

- After closed reduction, fit an extension gutter splint with the PIP joint in neutral position for continuous wear.

- The patient should perform active and passive ROM exercises of the MCP and DIP joints approximately 6 times a day.
- Do not allow PIP joint motion for 6 weeks.
- Begin active ROM exercises at 6 weeks in combination with intermittent daytime splinting and continuous night splinting for an additional 2 weeks.
- After open reduction and internal fixation of a dorsal marginal fracture, remove the transarticular pin between 2 and 4 weeks after the wound has healed, and ensure continuous splinting in an extension gutter splint for a total of 6 weeks. The remainder of the protocol is similar to that used after the closed technique.

▐ *Continue extension splinting as long as an extensor lag is present, and avoid passive flexion exercises as long as an extension lag of 30 degrees or more is present.*

Dorsal fracture-dislocations of the PIP joint are much more common than volar dislocations. If less than 50% of the articular surface is involved, these injuries usually are stable after a closed reduction and protective splinting in flexion.

- If the injury is believed to be stable after closed reduction, apply a DBS with the PIP joint in 30 degrees of flexion. This allows for full flexion but prevents the terminal 30 degrees of extension.
- After 3 weeks, adjust the DBS at weekly intervals to increase PIP extension by about 10 degrees each week.
- The splint should be in the neutral position by the sixth week and then discontinued.
- Begin an active ROM program and use dynamic extension splinting as needed.
- Begin progressive strengthening exercises at 8 weeks.

Dorsal fracture-dislocations involving more than 50% of the articular surface may be unstable, even with the digit in flexion, and may require surgical intervention. The Eaton volar plate advancement is probably the most common procedure used. The fracture fragments are excised, and the volar plate is advanced into the remaining portion of the middle phalanx. The PIP joint usually is pinned in 30 degrees of flexion.

- At 3 weeks after surgery, remove the pin from the PIP joint and fit a DBS with the PIP joint in 30 degrees of flexion for continuous wear.
- Begin active and active-assisted ROM exercises within the restraints of the DBS.
- At 5 weeks discontinue the DBS and continue active and passive extension exercises.

- At 6 weeks dynamic extension splinting may be necessary if full passive extension has not been regained.

Flexion contractures are not uncommon after this procedure. Agee described the use of an external fixator combined with rubber bands that allows early active ROM of the PIP joint in unstable fracture-dislocation while maintaining reduction. The bulky hand dressing is removed 3 to 5 days after surgery, and active ROM exercises are carried out for 10-minute sessions every 2 hours. Pins should be cleansed twice daily with the use of cotton swabs and hydrogen peroxide, protecting the base of the pin with gauze. The external fixator may be removed between 3 and 6 weeks. An unrestricted active and passive ROM exercise program is started.

Dorsal dislocations of the PIP joint without associated fractures usually are stable after closed reduction. Stability is tested after reduction under digital block and, if the joint is believed to be stable, buddy taping for 3 to 6 weeks, early active ROM exercises, and edema control are necessary. If instability is present with passive extension of the joint, a DBS, similar to that used in fracture-dislocations, should be used.

Intraarticular fractures involving the base of the thumb metacarpal are classified as either *Bennett fractures* (if a single volar ulnar fragment exists) or a *Rolando fracture* (if there is a T-condylar fracture pattern). These fractures often displace because of the proximal pull of the APL on the base of the proximal thumb metacarpal.

Nondisplaced Bennett fractures are treated in a short-arm thumb spica cast, which can be removed at 6 weeks if the fracture has healed clinically. Active and gentle passive ROM exercises are begun. At that time the patient is also fitted with a removable thumb spica splint. This should be used between exercise sessions and at night for an additional 2 weeks. Strengthening exercises are then started using silicone putty. The patient generally returns to normal activity between 10 and 12 weeks. If there is persistent joint subluxation after application of a short-arm cast with the thumb positioned in palmar and radial abduction, closed reduction and percutaneous pinning are carried out. After pinning, the thumb is placed in a thumb spica splint and protected for 6 weeks. After the pin is removed, therapy progresses as described for nondisplaced fractures.

Rolando fractures have poor prognoses. The choice of treatment usually depends on the severity of comminution and the degree of displacement. If large fragments are present with displacement, open reduction and internal fixation with Kirschner wires or a mini-fragment plate are performed. If severe comminution is present, manual molding in palmar abduction and immobilization in a thumb spica cast for 3 to 4 weeks are recommended. After stable internal fixation, motion may be started at 6 weeks in a manner similar to that for Bennett fractures.

REHABILITATION PROTOCOL

Nondisplaced Metacarpal Fracture

0 to 3 weeks	• Begin active PIP and DIP flexion and extension exercises. • Elevate hand for edema control. • Begin gentle active and active-assisted ROM exercises. • Begin strengthening exercises with silicone putty. • Continue exercises until grip strength is restored.
3 weeks	• Discontinue splinting. • Protect fingers with buddy taping.

REHABILITATION PROTOCOL

Postsurgical Metacarpal and Phalangeal Fractures

0 to 4 days	• Apply a bulky hand dressing with an anterior-posterior splint in the position of function. • If fixation is tenuous but alignment is adequate, immobilize the hand in the position of function for a full 3 weeks.
4 days	• Remove the splint and apply an anterior-posterior splint or a well-molded orthoplast splint that allows PIP and DIP motion. The MCP joint may be immobilized in flexion during this period.
3 to 6 weeks	• Begin active motion before pin removal.

INJURIES TO THE ULNAR COLLATERAL LIGAMENT OF THE THUMB METACARPOPHALANGEAL JOINT (GAMEKEEPER'S THUMB)

Injuries to the ulnar collateral ligament of the thumb MCP joint are common. They may be partial or complete ruptures of the ligament. Complete ruptures are called gamekeeper's thumb or skier's thumb and can be differentiated from partial tears by obtaining anterior-posterior (AP) stress views of the thumb MCP joint. If the thumb MCP joint angulates more than 30 degrees with radial directed stress compared with the uninjured side, the injury is considered a complete tear, and surgical intervention is indicated (see protocol, p. 62).

SCAPHOID FRACTURES

Nondisplaced scaphoid fractures are treated initially in a long-arm thumb spica cast for 6 weeks, followed by a short-arm spica cast for an additional 6 weeks until roentgenographic union is evident. Fractures involving the proximal and central portions of the scaphoid often require longer periods of immobilization. Active ROM exercises to the forearm, wrist, and thumb should be carried out 6 to 8 times daily after prolonged immobilization. A wrist and thumb static splint often is fitted with the wrist in neutral to be worn between exercise sessions and at night.

Displaced fractures usually require open reduction and internal fixation using either multiple Kirschner wires, a small cancellous screw, or a Herbert screw. Usually, the fracture is treated in a short-arm thumb spica splint until roentgenographic union is achieved, usually in 8 to 12 weeks. Occasionally, if good screw fixation is achieved (as determined by the surgeon intraoperatively), an extremely compliant patient may be treated initially in a short-arm splint for 3 to 4 weeks, followed by application of a removable orthoplast thumb spica splint to be worn during activity until there is roentgenographic evidence of a union. The splint should be removed only 3 times a day for gentle ROM exercises and for bathing. At 4 months after surgery, dynamic wrist flexion and extension may be initiated to increase passive wrist motion. Usually the patient is able to resume normal use of the hand without restriction by 6 months after surgery, provided ROM has been regained and union is evident on roentgenogram.

Ulnar Collateral Ligament (UCL) Strain of Thumb Metacarpophalangeal Joint

Mechanism:	Typically, a ski pole or gamekeeper's thumb type of mechanism, but *not an unstable injury* (only a strain), that can be treated nonoperatively.
0 to 3 weeks	• Fit opponens splint with thumb in palmar abduction; splint is worn continuously.
3 to 6 weeks	• Reevaluate stability and discomfort. • Begin active and gentle passive ROM exercises of thumb. • If ROM is unstable or painful, have physician reevaluate. • Patient should wear the splint for protection and comfort and remove it several times a day for exercise sessions.
8 weeks	• Patient should be asymptomatic. • Discontinue splint except for sports, heavy lifting, or repetitive pinching. • Use progressive strengthening exercises.

REHABILITATION PROTOCOL

Repair or Reconstruction of Ulnar Collateral Ligament of Thumb Metacarpophalangeal Joint*

Indications:	Typically after repair of gamekeeper's thumb.
3 weeks	• Remove bulky dressing. • Remove MCP pin if used for joint stabilization. • Fit with wrist and thumb static splint for continual wear.
6 weeks	• Begin active and gentle passive ROM exercises of thumb for 10 minutes each hour.

■ *Avoid any lateral stress to the MCP joint of the thumb.*

	• Begin dynamic splinting if necessary to increase passive ROM of thumb.
8 weeks	• Discontinue splinting. Wrist and thumb static splint or short opponens splint may be useful during sports-related activities or heavy lifting. • Begin progressive strengthening.
12 weeks	• Allow the patient to return to unrestricted activity.

COLLES' FRACTURES OF THE WRIST

Classification Systems

Frykman

- Even-numbered fractures (types II, IV, VI, and VIII) have an associated fracture of the distal ulna.
- Types III through VI are intraarticular fractures.
- Higher numbers in the classification have worse prognoses.
- Joint involvement

I, II	Extraarticular
III, IV	Radiocarpal joint
V, VI	Radioulnar joint
VII, VIII	Both radiocarpal and radioulnar joints

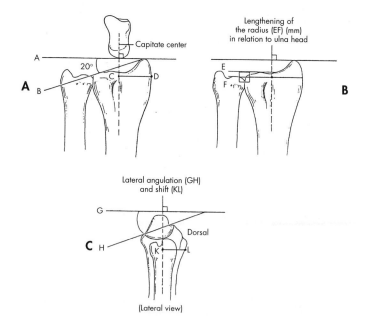

Figure 1-19 The location of lines to be drawn for measuring radial slope, radial length, and volar inclination of the distal radius are shown in **A, B,** and **C,** respectively. (From Putnam MD: *Fractures and dislocations of the carpus including the distal radius.* In Gustillo RB, Kyle RF, Templeman D, editors: *Fractures and dislocations,* St. Louis, 1993, Mosby–Year Book.)

Goals of Treatment

- Restoration of radial length (Fig. 1-19, *B*).
- Restoration of volar tilt (Fig. 1-19, *C*).
- Restoration of anatomic articular congruity.
- Avoidance of complications.
- Appropriate treatment with consideration of patient's physiologic age, functional demands, occupation, and handedness.
- Early motion of a stable construct.

Complications

- Stiff wrist and/or fingers
- Posttraumatic arthritis
- Residual deformity
- Reflex sympathetic dystrophy
- Malunion, nonunion, delayed union
- Transient or permanent neuropathy

Treatment Considerations

The algorithm described by Palmer bases treatment on physiologic age and demand, stability, displacement, articular congruity, shortening, and angulation (Table 1-2).

TABLE 1-2 Palmer Treatment Algorithm

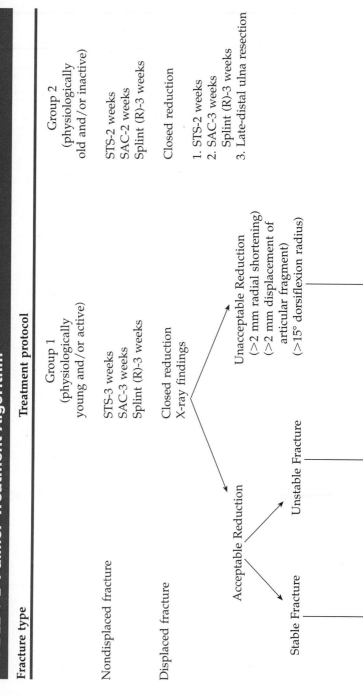

Fracture type	Treatment protocol		
	Group 1 (physiologically young and/or active)		Group 2 (physiologically old and/or inactive)
Nondisplaced fracture	STS-3 weeks SAC-3 weeks Splint (R)-3 weeks		STS-2 weeks SAC-2 weeks Splint (R)-3 weeks
Displaced fracture	Closed reduction X-ray findings		Closed reduction 1. STS-2 weeks 2. SAC-3 weeks Splint (R)-3 weeks 3. Late-distal ulna resection

Acceptable Reduction → Unstable Fracture, Stable Fracture

Unacceptable Reduction (>2 mm radial shortening) (>2 mm displacement of articular fragment) (>15° dorsiflexion radius)

STS-3 weeks
LAC-3 weeks
Splint (R)-3 weeks

1. External fixation
   with supplemental
   percutaneous pins
   Ex fix-6 weeks
   Pins-8 weeks
   Splint (R)-3 weeks

2. ORIF (plate)
   SAS-10 days
   Splint (R)-5 weeks

3. Percutaneous pins

   STS-3 weeks
   SAC-3 weeks
   Pins-6 weeks
   Splint (R)-3 weeks

1. External fixation with fragment
   elevation (pins optional) and
   iliac crest bone graft-5 weeks

2. ORIF (K-wire) with iliac crest bone graft
   Ex fix-6 weeks
   Pins-6 weeks
   SAS-6 weeks
   Splint (R)-4 weeks

Modified from Palmar AK: *Fractures of the distal radius*. In Green D: *Operative hand surgery*, ed 3, New York, 1993, Churchill Livingstone. Our protocol for the treatment of nondisplaced and displaced distal radial fractures in the physiologically young and/or active (group 1) and the physiologically old and/or inactive (group 2). Nondisplaced fractures are easily treated with immobilization alone in both groups. Displaced fractures require reduction in both groups, but only in group 1 do we recommend further treatment. Based on the reduction and whether the fracture is stable or not, immobilization is recommended with or without operative treatment. Fractures where the reduction is unacceptable require reduction of the fragments with external fixation and/or internal fixation and bone grafting. *R,* removable; *STS,* sugar tong splint; *SAC,* short-arm cast; *LAC,* long-arm cast; *SAS,* short arm splint.

REHABILITATION PROTOCOL

Stable Colles' Fracture*

1 day	• Use a sugar tong splint. • Ice for 72 hours. • Elevate in cradle boot or on pillows for 2 to 3 days at home. • Begin active and passive ROM exercises to thumb, digits, and shoulder to be performed 10 minutes each hour. • Use dynamic splinting of the thumb and/or digits 4 to 6 times a day as needed. • Begin edema control with coban or finger socks to the thumb and digits. ■ *Watch for increased levels of edema and pain, which may result in reflex sympathetic dystrophy.*
4 to 6 weeks	• Remove splint. • Fit wrist immobilization splint for continual wear or between exercises and at night (depending on radiographic evidence of healing of fracture).
	• Begin active ROM exercises to wrist and forearm for 10 minutes each hour (assuming the fracture is well healed). • If necessary, begin FES to thumb, digits, wrist, and forearm. • Continue edema control as needed.
6 to 8 weeks	• Begin passive ROM exercises to wrist and forearm, 10 minutes each hour: flexion, extension, supination, and pronation. • If needed, begin dynamic splinting of wrist and/or forearm 4 to 6 times a day. • Decrease or discontinue wrist immobilization splint as comfort permits. • Begin progressive strengthening as needed. • Joint mobilization may help to improve ROM of the wrist and forearm, but is indicated *only* if the fracture is well healed on radiograph.

REHABILITATION PROTOCOL

Colles' Fracture Treated With External Fixation*

1 day	• Ice for 72 hours. • Elevate in cradle boot or pillows for 72 hours. • Perform routine neurovascular checks.
3 days	• Remove bulky compressive dressing and apply light compressive dressing evenly and carefully around pins. • Clean pin tracts twice a day with hydrogen peroxide and sterile cotton swab. • Apply gauze at base of pins to absorb drainage and prevent infection. • Begin active ROM and gentle passive ROM to fingers, elbow, shoulder, and thumb. Apply passive forearm rotation proximal to the fracture site only within the comfort level of the patient.
	• It usually is necessary to concentrate on passive motion of the thumb and index finger because of the proximity of the fixator pins to the EPL and extensor indicis pollicis (EIP)/extensor digitorum communis (EDC).
6 to 8 weeks	• Remove fixator (dependent on healing). • Begin active ROM exercises of wrist and forearm 10 minutes each hour. • Continue wrist immobilization splint at night and between exercise sessions for protection. • Begin strengthening with putty and/or hand exercise.

Continued

REHABILITATION PROTOCOL—cont'd

Colles' Fracture Treated With External Fixation*

8 to 10 weeks	• Begin passive ROM exercises to wrist (if fracture is healed). • Begin dynamic splinting of wrist as necessary. • Begin gentle progressive resistive exercises of wrist.

Advantages of External Fixation Include the Following:

- Supplementation of internal fixation that is maintaining articular alignment.
- Maintenance of length of radius to avoid fracture settling.
- Alleviation of compressive load forces to the wrist.
- Early forearm ROM and unrestricted active and passive ROM of digits and thumb.

CHAPTER TWO

Elbow Rehabilitation

JAMES R. ANDREWS, MD
KEVIN E. WILK, PT
DAVID GROH, PT

Elbow Dislocation

REHABILITATION RATIONALE

Elbow dislocations most frequently occur as a result of hyperextension, in which the olecranon process is forced into the olecranon fossa with such impact that the trochlea is levered over the coronoid process. Most elbow dislocations occur in a directly posterior or posterolateral direction.

Classification

The traditional classification of elbow dislocations divides injuries into anterior and posterior dislocations. Posterior dislocations are further subdivided according to the final resting position of the olecranon in relation to the distal humerus: posterior, posterolateral (most common), posteromedial (least common), or pure lateral.

Many elbow dislocations are accompanied by some type of ulnar collateral ligament (UCL) involvement. Repair of this ligament is sometimes indicated in athletes if the injury occurs in the dominant arm. This optimizes the chance for full return to the athlete's previous level of competition.

GENERAL REHABILITATION CONSIDERATIONS

▪ *The most common sequela of elbow dislocations is the loss of motion, especially extension.*

At 10 weeks, a flexion contracture averaging 30 degrees is common, and at 2 years a 10-degree flexion contracture often is present. This condition does not improve with time.

Rehabilitation is focused on restoring early range of motion (ROM) within the limits of elbow stability. *Valgus stress* to the elbow is *avoided* during rehabilitation.

Stability after reduction of an elbow dislocation must be determined to ensure proper rehabilitation. The elbow is moved through a gentle passive ROM, avoiding any valgus stressing. Redislocation of the elbow with simple passive ROM implies severe valgus instability with rupture of the medial collateral ligaments and forearm flexors.

For dislocations that are *stable* after reduction, best results are obtained with early protected motion before 2 weeks. Prolonged immobilization (more than 2 weeks) is associated with more severe flexion contracture and more pain at follow-up, and it does not decrease symptoms of instability. Stable elbow dislocations are effectively treated with early ROM and general strengthening, as with other rehabilitation protocols for the elbow. Inherent osseous stability allows early extension and flexion if valgus stress is prevented after reduction.

Unstable dislocations require repair of the medial collateral ligament. Rehabilitation of unstable dislocations requires a longer protection phase. Starting at week 1, a ROM brace preset at 30 to 90 degrees is implemented. Each week, motion in this brace is increased by 5 degrees of extension and 10 degrees of flexion. This progression is controlled directly by the collagen synthesis and remodeling process that takes place within the involved tissues.

A rehabilitation program that is too aggressive may cause recurrent subluxation, and one that is too conservative can lead to a flexion contracture; the occurrence of flexion contractures is a much greater probability. Full elbow extension is less critical for the nonathlete and thus may be sacrificed slightly to ensure that the joint structure and ligaments are given more time to heal and to decrease the risk of recurrent subluxation or dislocation.

REHABILITATION PROTOCOL

Stable Elbow Dislocation   ANDREWS AND WILK

1 to 4 days	• Immobilize the elbow in a posterior splint for 3 to 4 days. • Begin light gripping exercises. • Begin active ROM in all planes. • Begin shoulder isometrics. Avoid valgus stress to the elbow. • Use pulsed ultrasound and high-voltage galvanic stimulation (HVGS) modalities as required.
5 to 9 days	• The splint should be removed for exercises. • Begin gentle active ROM exercises of elbow out of the splint several times a day but no passive ROM. • Begin active ROM in elbow flexion/extension, supination/pronation, and slow Upper Body Ergonometer (UBE). • Begin isometrics in elbow flexion/extension at varying angles. • Begin shoulder strength progression with stabilization of elbow; begin wrist isotonics.
10 to 14 days	• Discard the splint. • Continue active ROM exercises. • Initiate full elbow rehabilitation program, including passive ROM. • Begin progressive resistance exercises as tolerated for elbow; begin supination and pronation also. • Perform isotonic exercises; use caution with external rotation (ER) to avoid valgus stress to the elbow. • A hinged brace may be used and locked from 15 to 90 degrees for up to 4 weeks if borderline stability is a concern.
Return to sports	• Do not allow return to participation in sports until strength, power, and endurance is 85% to 90% of the uninvolved limb. • Brace is worn and locked on parameters to prevent elbow hyperextension and valgus stress once the athlete returns to competition.

REHABILITATION PROTOCOL

Unstable Elbow Dislocation ANDREWS AND WILK

Phase 1—Immediate Postreduction Phase

0 to 3 weeks
- Goals:
  Protect healing tissue.
  Decrease pain/inflammation.
  Retard muscular atrophy.
- Set splint or brace ROM at 10 degrees less than active ROM elbow extension limit.
- Perform elbow flexion to patient tolerance.
- Perform wrist active ROM flexion/extension and supination/pronation exercises, 5 degrees of extension and 10 degrees of flexion per week (as long as there is no associated fracture).
- *Avoid any varus/valgus stress on the elbow.*
- Initiate further exercises:
  Gripping exercises.
  Wrist ROM.

Shoulder "straight plane isometrics" (no shoulder internal rotation [IR] or ER); biceps multiangle isometrics.
- Use cryotherapy.
- Use pulsed ultrasound or HVGS.

Phase 2—Intermediate Phase

4 to 8 weeks
- Goals:
  Gradual increase in elbow extension ROM (10 degrees per week).
  Promote healing of damaged tissue.
  Regain and improve muscle strength.

4 weeks
- Set functional brace at 10 degrees greater than it was in the previous week.
- Begin light resistance exercises for arm (1 lb).
  Wrist curls, extensions.

Continued

REHABILITATION PROTOCOL—cont'd

Unstable Elbow Dislocation ANDREWS AND WILK

Phase 2—Intermediate Phase—cont'd

4 weeks —cont'd	Pronation/supination. Elbow flexion/extension. • Progress shoulder program. Emphasize rotator cuff strengthening (avoid IR/ER until the sixth week). • Begin gentle passive ROM for elbow flexion/extension.
6 weeks	• Progress elbow strengthening exercises. • Initiate shoulder ER strengthening. • Progress shoulder program.

Phase 3—Advanced Strengthening Phase

9 to 13 weeks	• Goals: Increase strength, power, endurance. Maintain full elbow ROM. Gradually initiate sports activities.
9 weeks	• Initiate eccentric elbow flexion/extension. • Continue isotonic program for forearm and wrist. • Continue shoulder program (Thrower's Ten Program, p. 89). • Begin manual resistance diagonal patterns. • Initiate plyometric exercise program.
11 weeks	• Continue all exercises. • Patient may begin light sports activities (such as golf and swimming).

Lateral and Medial Epicondylitis

REHABILITATION RATIONALE

Classic lateral epicondylitis (tennis elbow) is caused by repetitive microtrauma that results in degeneration of the extensor carpi radialis brevis tendon. Repetitive eccentric muscle overload has been implicated in the development of lateral epicondylitis. A change in the patient's regular activity or an overuse syndrome should be sought in the history as a precipitating cause.

Mechanism

Lateral Epicondylitis. In tennis players, improper backhand stroke and wrist extension or flipping of the wrist may produce an overuse extensor tendonitis, especially of the extensor carpi radialis brevis muscle (Fig. 2-1). Serving with the racquet in pronation and snapping the wrist to impart spin also may cause lateral epicondylitis. Activities involving repetitive use of the extensor wad other than tennis may cause lateral epicondylitis.

Medial Epicondylitis. "Golfer's elbow" is produced in the right elbow in a right-handed golf swing by throwing the club head down at the ball with the right arm rather than pulling the club through with the left arm and trunk. This unorthodox swing causes stress at the flexor pronator group. Symptoms of medial epicondylitis include pain at the muscle group origin with resisted wrist flexion, pronation, or both. Weakness, commonly a result of pain, also may be detected in grasping activities.

General Rehabilitation Considerations

A general outline of rehabilitation includes *gentle stretching exercises* initiated through wrist flexion, extension, and rotation (Fig. 2-2). These are held for 10 seconds and repeated for 5 to 10 repetitions. Vigorous stretching is avoided until the patient is pain free.

When the injury results from eccentric overload, *eccentric strengthening* is important to prevent recurrence (Fig. 2-3, *A*). Re-

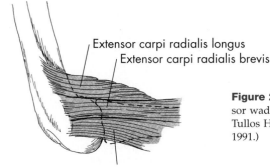

Extensor carpi radialis longus
Extensor carpi radialis brevis

Figure 2-1 Lateral extensor wad. (Redrawn from Tullos H: *Instr Course Lect,* 1991.)

Extensor digitorum communis

sistive training includes wrist flexion and extension in addition to forearm pronation and supination. This should be in a pain-free range (Figs. 2-3, *B-E,* and 2-4).

Equipment modifications that may be helpful include increasing the grip size of a racquet, decreasing string tension, and choosing a racquet with good vibration absorption characteristics (graphite, ceramic, composites). There is some disagreement on grip size in the literature, and recent studies have suggested that grip size may be less important than previously thought.

Lateral counterforce bracing is believed to diminish the magnitude of muscle contraction, decreasing muscle tension in the region of the damaged musculocutaneous unit. Counterforce bracing should be used as a supplement to, not a replacement for, muscular strengthening exercises.

Epicondylitis is a common and often lingering pathologic condition. For this reason, it is critical that the rehabilitation process is progressed with minimal or no pain. The stressful components of high-level activity usually can be alleviated by altering the frequency, intensity, or duration of play.

Galloway, DeMaio, and Mangine also divide their approach to patients with epicondylitis (medial or lateral) into three stages:

- The initial phase is directed toward reducing inflammation, preparing the patient for phase 2.
- The second phase emphasizes return of strength and endurance. Specific inciting factors are identified and modified.
- Phase 3 involves functional rehabilitation designed to return the patient to the desired activity level.

This protocol is also based on the severity of the initial symptoms and objective findings at initiation treatment.

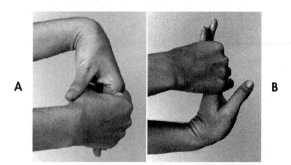

Figure 2-2 **A,** Wrist extensor stretching. Grasp the hand and slowly flex the wrist down until sustained stretch is felt. Hold for 10 seconds. Repeat 5 times per session, several times a day. **B,** Wrist flexor stretching. Grasp the hand and slowly extend the wrist until a sustained stretch is felt. Hold for 10 seconds. Repeat 5 times per session, several times a day.

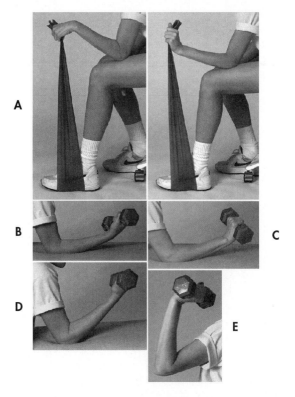

Figure 2-3 A, Eccentric wrist extension exercises with rubber band. **B**, Wrist flexion-resistive training. **C**, Wrist extension-resistive training. **D**, Elbow flexion-resisitive training. **E**, Elbow extension-resistive training.

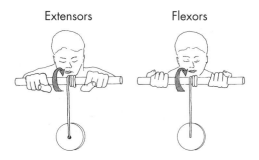

Figure 2-4 Wrist flexors and extensors. The patient rolls up a string with a weight tied on the end. The weight may be progressively increased. Flexors are worked with the palms up, extensors with the palms down. (From Galloway M, DeMaio M, Mangine R: Rehabilitative techniques in the treatment of medial and lateral epicondylitis, *Orthopedics* 15(9):1089, 1992.)

REHABILITATION PROTOCOL

Epicondylitis   WILK AND ANDREWS

Phase 1—Acute Phase

- Goals:
  Decrease inflammation/pain.
  Promote tissue healing.
  Retard muscular atrophy.
- Cryotherapy.
- Whirlpool.
- Stretching to increase flexibility.
  Wrist extension/flexion.
  Elbow extension/flexion.
  Forearm supination/pronation.
- Isometrics
  Wrist extension/flexion.
  Elbow extension/flexion.
  Forearm supination/pronation.

Phase 2—Subacute Phase

- Goals:
  Improve flexibility.
  Increase muscular strength and endurance.
  Increase functional activities and return to function.
- Emphasize concentric/eccentric strengthening.
  Concentrate on involved muscle group(s).
  Wrist extension/flexion (see Fig. 2-6, A).
  Forearm pronation/supination.
  Elbow flexion/extension.
- Initiate shoulder strengthening (if deficiencies are noted).

Phase 3—Chronic Phase

- Goals:
  Improve muscular strength and endurance.
  Maintain/enhance flexibility.
  Gradually return to sport/high-level activities.
- Continue strengthening exercises (emphasize eccentric/concentric).
- Continue to emphasize deficiencies in shoulder and elbow strength.
- Continue flexibility exercises.
- Gradually diminish use of counterforce brace.

Phase 1—Acute Phase—cont'd
- HVGS.
- Phonophoresis.
- Friction massage.
- Iontophoresis (with an antiinflammatory such as dexamethasone).
- Avoid painful movements (such as gripping).

Phase 2—Subacute Phase—cont'd
- Continue flexibility exercises.
- May use counterforce brace.
- Continue use of cryotherapy after exercise or function.
- Initiate gradual return to stressful activities.
- Gradually reinitiate previously painful movements.

Phase 3—Chronic Phase—cont'd
- Use cryotherapy as needed.
- Initiate gradual return to sport activity.
- Equipment modifications (grip size, string tension, playing surface).
- Emphasize maintenance program.

REHABILITATION PROTOCOL

Evaluation-Based Rehabilitation Medial and Lateral Epicondylitis
GALLOWAY, DE MAIO, AND MANGINE

Rationale: Patients begin a rehabilitation protocol based on their symptoms and objective physical findings. The initial phase of each protocol is directed toward restoring ROM at the wrist and elbow. Phase 2 involves strength training and a structured return to activity.

	Protocol 1 (Severe Symptoms)	Protocol 2 (Mild/Moderate Symptoms)	Protocol 3 (Symptoms Resolved)
When	• Pain at rest • Point tenderness • Pain with minimally resisted wrist extension • Swelling • Grip strength difference (GSD) >50% • >5° motion loss at wrist/elbow	• Pain with activity only • Minimal point tenderness • Minimal pain with resisted wrist flexion/extension • GSD >50% • No motion loss	• No pain with daily activity • No referred pain • Full ROM • GSD <10%
Evaluation	• Duration of symptoms • Referred pain • Grip strength measurement • Elbow palpation • Motion measurement • History of injury or inciting activity • Differential diagnosis	• Duration of symptoms • Referred pain • Grip strength measurement • Elbow palpation • Motion measurement • History of injury or inciting activity • Differential diagnosis	• Review initial injury or inciting activity • Identify requirements for returning to desired activity • Identify remaining functional deficits

Treatment	Phase 1 (Reduced Inflammation)	Phase 1 (Reduce Inflammation)	Preactivity flexibility
	• Rest	• Rest	• Strengthening
	• Passive ROM	• Passive ROM	-isokinetic
	• Cold therapy	• Cold therapy	-isotonic
	• Medications	• Medications	• Modalities
			-whirlpool
			-ice after activity
	Phase 2 (Rehabilitation)	Phase 2 (Rehabilitation)	• Technique modification
	• Limit activity	• Limit activity	• Equipment modification
	• Cold therapy	• Flexibility	• Counterforce bracing
	• Stretching (static)	• Strengthening	• Friction massage
	• Strengthening (isometric)	• Transverse friction massage	• Gradual return to activity
	• Ultrasound	• Cold therapy	
	• HVGS	• HVGS	
	• Proceed to Protocol 2 when tolerating above	• Ultrasound	
	• Surgical indications	• Proceed to Protocol 3	
Goals	• Resolution of pain at rest	• No pain with daily activity	• Pain-free return to activity
	• Tolerate stretching/strengthening with minimal discomfort	• No pain with stretching/progressive resistance exercises (PREs)	• Prevent recurrence—maintenance program of stretching
	• Improve ROM	• Full ROM	
	• Maintain cardiovascular conditioning	• Prepare for functional rehabilitation	
		• Maintain cardiovascular conditioning	

Rehabilitation of the Elbow in Throwing Athletes

REHABILITATION RATIONALE

Slocum was one of the first to classify throwing injuries of the elbow into medial tension and valgus compression overload injuries.

■ *Valgus stress plus forced extension is the major pathologic mechanism of the thrower's elbow.*

Tension is produced on the medial aspect of the elbow. *Compression* is produced on the lateral aspect of the elbow. See the box for classification of these throwing injuries.

Elbow rehabilitation in throwing athletes generally follows a four-phase progression. It is important that certain criteria be met at each level before advancement is made to the next stage. This allows athletes to progress at their own pace based on tissue-healing constraints.

Phase 1 involves regaining motion lost during postsurgical immobilization. Pain, inflammation, and muscle atrophy also are treated.

Common regimens for inflammation and pain involve modalities such as cryotherapy, HVGS, ultrasound, and whirlpool. Joint mobilization techniques also can be used to help minimize pain and promote motion.

Classification of Injuries of the Elbow in Throwing Athletes

Medial Stress
- Flexor muscle strain or tear.
- Avulsion of medial epicondyle.
- Attenuation or tear of the medial collateral ligament.
- Ulnar nerve traction.

Lateral Compression
- Hypertrophy of the radial head and capitellum.
- Avascular necrosis of the capitellum.
- Osteochondral fractures of the radial head or capitellum.

Forced Extension
- Olecranon osteophyte formation on the tip of the olecranon process.
- Loose body formation.
- Scarring and fibrous tissue deposition in the olecranon fossa.

To minimize muscular atrophy, submaximal isometric exercises for elbow flexors and extensors, as well as for the forearm pronators and supinators, are started early. Strengthening of the shoulder also should begin relatively early to prevent functional weakness. Care should be taken early in the rehabilitation program to restrict ER movements that may place valgus stress on the medial structures of the elbow.

Elbow flexion contracture is common after an elbow injury or surgery when ROM is not treated appropriately. Prevention of these contractures is the key. Early ROM is vital to nourish the articular cartilage and promote proper collagen fiber alignment. A gradual increase in and early restoration of full passive elbow extension are essential to prevent flexion contraction. Several popular techniques to improve limited ROM are joint mobilization, contract-relax stretching, and low-load, long-duration stretching for the restoration of full elbow extension.

Joint mobilizations can be performed to the humeroulnar, humeroradial, and radioulnar joints. Limited elbow extension tends to respond to posterior glides of the ulna on the humerus.

Another technique to restore full elbow extension is *low-load, long-duration stretching.* A good passive overpressure stretch can be achieved by having the patient hold a 2- to 4-lb weight or use an elastic band with the upper extremity resting on a fulcrum just proximal to the elbow joint to allow for greater extension. This stretch should be performed for 10 to 12 minutes to incorporate a long-duration, low-intensity stretch. Stretching of this magnitude has been found to elicit a plastic collagen tissue response, resulting in permanent soft tissue elongation. It is important to note that if the intensity of this stretch is too great, pain and/or a protective muscle response may result, which could inhibit collagen fiber elongation.

Phase 2, or the "intermediate phase," consists of improving the patient's overall strength, endurance, and elbow mobility. To progress to this phase, the patient must demonstrate full elbow ROM (0 to 135 degrees), minimal or no pain or tenderness, and a "good" (4/5) muscle grade for the elbow flexor and extensor groups. During this phase, isotonic strengthening exercises are emphasized for the entire arm and shoulder complex.

Phase 3 is the advanced strengthening phase. The primary goal in this phase is to prepare the athlete for the return to functional participation and initiation of throwing activities. A total arm-strengthening program is used to improve the power, endurance, and neuromuscular control of the entire limb. Advancement to phase 3 requires demonstration of full, pain-free ROM, no pain or tenderness, and 70% strength compared to the contralateral side.

Interval Throwing Program
PHASE 1

45-Foot Phase

Step 1: A. Warm-up throwing
B. 45 feet (25 throws)
C. Rest 15 minutes
D. Warm-up throwing
E. 45 feet (25 throws)

Step 2: A. Warm-up throwing
B. 45 feet (25 throws)
C. Rest 10 minutes
D. Warm-up throwing
E. 45 feet (25 throws)
F. Rest 10 minutes
G. Warm-up throwing
H. 45 feet (25 throws)

60-Foot Phase

Step 3: A. Warm-up throwing
B. 60 feet (25 throws)
C. Rest 15 minutes
D. Warm-up throwing
E. 60 feet (25 throws)

Step 4: A. Warm-up throwing
B. 60 feet (25 throws)
C. Rest 10 minutes
D. Warm-up throwing
E. 60 feet (25 throws)
F. Rest 10 minutes
G. Warm-up throwing
H. 60 feet (25 throws)

90-Foot Phase

Step 5: A. Warm-up throwing
B. 90 feet (25 throws)
C. Rest 15 minutes
D. Warm-up throwing
E. 90 feet (25 throws)

Step 6: A. Warm-up throwing
B. 90 feet (25 throws)
C. Rest 10 minutes
D. Warm-up throwing
E. 90 feet (25 throws)
F. Rest 10 minutes
G. Warm-up throwing
H. 90 feet (25 throws)

120-Foot Phase

Step 7: A. Warm-up throwing
B. 120 feet (25 throws)
C. Rest 15 minutes
D. Warm-up throwing
E. 120 feet (25 throws)

Step 8: A. Warm-up throwing
B. 120 feet (25 throws)
C. Rest 10 minutes
D. Warm-up throwing
E. 120 feet (25 throws)
F. Rest 10 minutes
G. Warm-up throwing
H. 120 feet (25 throws)

150-Foot Phase

Step 9: A. Warm-up throwing
B. 150 feet (25 throws)
C. Rest 15 minutes
D. Warm-up throwing
E. 150 feet (25 throws)

Step 10: A. Warm-up throwing
B. 150 feet (25 throws)
C. Rest 10 minutes
D. Warm-up throwing
E. 150 feet (25 throws)
F. Rest 10 minutes
G. Warm-up throwing
H. 150 feet (25 throws)

180-Foot Phase

Step 11: A. Warm-up throwing
B. 180 feet (25 throws)
C. Rest 15 minutes
D. Warm-up throwing
E. 180 feet (25 throws)

Step 12: A. Warm-up throwing
B. 180 feet (25 throws)
C. Rest 10 minutes
D. Warm-up throwing
E. 180 feet (25 throws)
F. Rest 10 minutes
G. Warm-up throwing
H. 180 feet (25 throws)

Step 13: A. Warm-up throwing
B. 180 feet (25 throws)
C. Rest 10 minutes
D. Warm-up throwing
E. 180 feet (25 throws)
F. Rest 10 minutes
G. Warm-up throwing
H. 180 feet (25 throws)

Step 14: Begin throwing off the mound or return to respective position

Interval Throwing Program
PHASE 2

Stage 1: Fastball Only

Step 1: Interval throwing
   15 throws off mound 50%
Step 2: Interval throwing
   30 throws off mound 50%
Step 3: Interval throwing
   45 throws off mound 50%
Step 4: Interval throwing
   60 throws off mound 50%
Step 5: Interval throwing
   30 throws off mound 75%
Step 6: 30 throws off mound 75%
   45 throws off mound 50%
Step 7: 45 throws off mound 75%
   15 throws off mound 50%
Step 8: 60 throws off mound 75%

Stage 2: Fastball Only

Step 9: 45 throws off mound 75%
   15 throws in batting practice

Step 10: 45 throws off mound 75%
   30 throws in batting practice
Step 11: 45 throws off mound 75%
   45 throws in batting practice

Stage 3

Step 12: 30 throws off mound 75%
   warm-up
   15 throws off mound 50%
   breaking balls
Step 13: 30 throws off mound 75%
   30 breaking balls 75%
   30 throws in batting practice
Step 14: 30 throws off mound 75%
   60 to 90 throws in batting practice
   25% breaking balls
Step 15: Simulated game: progressing by 15 throws per work-
   out

Use interval throwing to 120-foot phase as a warm-up. All throwing off the mound should be done in the presence of the pitching coach to stress proper throwing mechanics. Use a speed gun to aid in effort control.

Plyometric exercises are most beneficial in this phase; these drills closely simulate functional activities, such as throwing and swinging, and are performed at higher speeds. Plyometrics use a stretch-shortening cycle of muscle, thus using eccentric/concentric muscle extension.

The primary targets for strengthening in this phase are the biceps, triceps, and wrist flexor/pronator muscles. The biceps, the wrist flexors, and pronators greatly reduce valgus stresses on the elbow during the throwing motion. Other key muscle groups stressed in this phase include the triceps and rotator cuff. The triceps are used in the acceleration phase of the throwing motion, while attention to the rotator cuff helps to establish the goal of total arm strengthening.

To improve shoulder strength, the throwing athlete is introduced to a set of known as the "Thrower's Ten" program (Table 2-1.)

■ *Rehabilitation of an injured elbow is different from any other rehabilitation program for throwing athletes. Initially, elbow extension ROM must be obtained to prevent elbow flexion contracture. Next, valgus stress needs to be minimized through the conditioning of elbow and wrist flexors, as well as the pronator muscle group. Finally, the shoulder, especially the rotator cuff musculature, must be included in the rehabilitation process. The rotator cuff is vital to the throwing pattern and, if not strengthened, can lead to future shoulder problems.*

Phase 4, the final stage of the rehabilitation program for the throwing athlete, is "return to activity." This stage uses a progressive interval throwing program (see the box) to gradually increase the demands on the upper extremity by controlling throwing distance, frequency, and duration.

TABLE 2-1 **"Thrower's Ten" Program**

1. Dumbbell exercises for the deltoid and supraspinatus musculature.
2. Prone horizontal shoulder abduction.
3. Prone shoulder extension.
4. IR at 90 degrees of abduction of the shoulder with tubing.
5. ER at 90 degrees of abduction of the shoulder with tubing.
6. Elbow flexion/extension exercises (exercise tubing).
7. Serratus anterior strengthening—progressive push-ups.
8. Diagonal D2 pattern for shoulder flexion and extension with exercise tubing.
9. Press-ups.
10. Dumbbell wrist extension/flexion and pronation/supination.

REHABILITATION PROTOCOL

Isolated Subcutaneous Ulnar Nerve Transposition   WILK AND ANDREWS

Phase 1—Immediate Postoperative Phase

- Goals:
  Allow soft tissue healing of relocated nerve.
  Decrease pain and inflammation.
  Retard muscular atrophy.

1 week

- Posterior splint at 90 degrees of elbow flexion with wrist free for motion (sling for comfort).
- Compression dressing.
- Exercises: gripping exercises, wrist ROM, shoulder isometrics.

2 weeks

- Remove posterior splint for exercise and bathing.
- Progress elbow ROM (passive ROM 15 to 120 degrees).
- Initiate elbow and wrist isometrics.
- Continue shoulder isometrics.

Phase 2—Intermediate Phase

- Goals:
  Restore full pain-free ROM.
  Improve strength, power, endurance of upper extremity musculature.
  Gradually increase functional demands.

3 weeks

- Discontinue posterior splint.
- Progress elbow ROM, emphasize full extension.
- Initiate flexibility exercises for wrist extension/flexion, forearm supination/pronation, elbow extension/flexion.
- Initiate strengthening exercises for wrist extension/flexion, forearm supination/pronation, elbow extensors/flexors, shoulder program.

Phase 2—Intermediate Phase—cont'd

6 weeks
- Continue all exercises listed above.
- Initiate light sport activities.

Phase 3—Advanced Strengthening Phase
- Goals:
  Increase strength, power, and endurance.
  Gradually initiate sports activities.

8 weeks
- Initiate eccentric exercise program.
- Initiate plyometric exercise drills.

- Continue shoulder and elbow strengthening and flexibility exercises.
- Initiate interval throwing program.

Phase 4—Return to Activity Phase
- Goals:
  Gradually return to sports activities.

12 weeks
- Return to competitive throwing.
- Continue Thrower's Ten exercise program (see p. 89).

Arthroplasty (Posterior Decompression) of the Elbow

The most common indication for arthroscopic elbow posterior decompression arthroplasty is the presence of a posterior compartment osteophyte, which often is caused by valgus extension overload activities, such as throwing a baseball. The primary goal after arthroplasty, as after any arthroscopic elbow procedure, is to reestablish full elbow and wrist ROM as soon as possible. Motion should be at least 15 to 90 degrees 10 days after surgery, reaching 10 to 100 degrees at 2 weeks. By 20 to 25 days after surgery, the patient should have full ROM of the elbow.

REHABILITATION PROTOCOL

Elbow Arthroplasty (Posterior Compartment/Valgus Extension Overload)

Phase 1—Immediate Motion Phase

- Goals:
  Improve motion, regain full ROM.
  Decrease pain and inflammation.
  Retard muscular atrophy.

1 to 4 days	• Perform ROM to tolerance (extension/flexion and supination/pronation). Often full elbow extension is not possible because of pain.
	• Use gentle overpressure into extension.
	• Begin wrist flexion/extension stretches.
	• Begin gripping exercises (putty).
	• Begin isometrics: Wrist extensors/flexors. Elbow extensors/flexors.
5 to 10 days	• Use compression dressing, ice 4 to 5 times daily.
	• Perform ROM exercises to tolerance (at least 20 to 90 degrees).
	• Use overpressure into extension.
	• Use joint mobilization to reestablish ROM.
	• Continue wrist flexion/extension stretches.
	• Continue isometrics.
	• Continue use of ice and compression to control swelling.
11 to 14 days	• Perform ROM exercises to tolerance (at least 10 to 100 degrees).
	• Use overpressure into extension (3 to 4 times daily).
	• Continue joint mobilization techniques.

Continued

REHABILITATION PROTOCOL—cont'd

Elbow Arthroplasty (Posterior Compartment/Valgus Extension Overload)

Phase 1—Immediate Motion Phase—cont'd	• Initiate shoulder program (especially external rotators, rotator cuff).
11 to 14 days—cont'd	• Initiate light dumbbell program (PREs) biceps, triceps. Wrist flexors/extensors, supinators/pronators. • Continue joint mobilization. • Continue use of ice after exercise.
	• Continue use of ice after exercise.
Phase 2—Intermediate Phase	• Continue all exercises listed above.
4 to 7 weeks	• Goal: Improve strength, power, and endurance.
	• Initiate light upper body program. • Continue use of ice after activity.
2 to 4 weeks	• Perform full ROM exercises (4 to 5 times daily). • Use overpressure into elbow extension. • Continue PRE program for elbow and wrist musculature.
Phase 3—Advanced Strengthening Program.	• Goals: Improve strength, power, and endurance.
8 to 12 weeks	• Gradually return to functional activities. • Criteria to begin phase 3: Full nonpainful ROM. Strength at least 75% of contralateral side. No pain or tenderness.
	• Continue PRE program for elbow and wrist. • Continue shoulder program. • Continue stretching for elbow and shoulder. • Initiate interval program and gradual return to sports activities.

REHABILITATION PROTOCOL

Elbow Arthroscopy

Phase 1—Immediate Motion Phase

1 to 2 days

- Goals:
  Regain full, pain-free wrist and elbow ROM.
  Decrease pain and inflammation.
  Retard muscular atrophy.
- Remove bulky dressing; replace with elastic dressing.
- Initiate wrist and elbow ROM exercises.
- Initiate putty/gripping exercises.
- Begin flexibility exercises: wrist extension/flexion, supination/pronation.
- Begin elbow active ROM and active-assisted ROM (motion to tolerance).
- Begin isometric strengthening exercises (shoulder, elbow, and wrist).

3 to 7 days

- Continue active ROM, and active-assisted ROM elbow (full ROM at day 7).
- Begin isotonic strengthening for wrist and elbow musculature (1 lb).

8 to 14 days

- Continue all exercises listed above.
- Continue ROM (0 to 125 degrees); emphasize full elbow extension.

Phase 2—Intermediate Phase

3 weeks

- Goals:
  Improve muscular strength, power, and endurance.
  Normalize joint arthrokinematics.
- Initiate elbow eccentric strengthening program.
- Initiate shoulder strengthening exercises.
- Continue ROM exercises for elbow.

Continued

REHABILITATION PROTOCOL—cont'd

Elbow Arthroscopy

Phase 3—Advanced Strengthening Phase
- Goals:
  Continue to increase strength and endurance.
  Prepare athlete for gradual return to functional activities.
- Criteria to progress to advanced phase:
  Full, nonpainful ROM.
  No pain or tenderness.
  Isokinetic test that fulfills criteria to throw.
  Satisfactory clinical exam.

5 weeks
- Continue all strengthening and flexibility exercises (Thrower's Ten Program, p. 89).
- Initiate interval throwing (phase 1, p. 88).

Phase 4—Return to Activity Phase
- Goals:
  Gradually return to functional activities.
  Continue strengthening exercises for upper extremity.

7 weeks
- Initiate competitive sports activities.
- Continue Thrower's Ten Program.
- Continue flexibility exercises (especially elbow extension stretches).
- Continue forearm supination/pronation.
- Continue all wrist/elbow exercises.

Isolated Fracture of the Radial Head

Mason's classification of radial head fractures is the most widely accepted and useful for treatment (Fig. 2-5). Rehabilitation is based on this classification (Table 2-2).

TABLE 2-2 **Mason's Classification of Radial Head Fractures**

Type	Description
Type I	Nondisplaced fracture Often missed on radiograph Positive posterior fat pad sign
Type II	Marginal radial head fractures with displacement, depression, or angulation
Type III	Comminuted fracture of the entire head
Type IV	Concomitant dislocation of elbow or other associated injuries

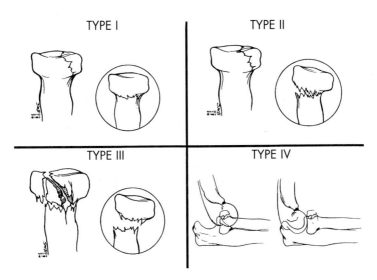

Figure 2-5 Mason classification of radial head fractures. (From Broberg MA, Morrey BF: Results of treatment of fracture dislocations of the elbow, *Clin Orthop* 216:109, 1987.)

TREATMENT

Nondisplaced type I fractures require little or no immobilization. Active and passive ROM may be begun immediately after injury to promote full ROM. Conditioning in the form of elbow flexion and extension, supination and pronation isometrics, and wrist and shoulder isotonics can be implemented immediately (usually within the first week) after injury. Stress to the radial head is minimized. Three to 6 weeks of active elbow flexion and extension may be used, along with wrist isotonics.

Types II and III fractures usually require open reduction internal fixation. Frequently, immobilization is required for a brief time, followed by active and passive ROM exercises.

Type IV comminuted fractures frequently require stabilization of the elbow joint and excision of fragments and usually cause some functional limitation. Full ROM rarely returns and chronic elbow pain often persists.

Treatment for types I, II, III, and IV fractures is described in Table 2-3.

TABLE 2-3 Treatment of Radial Head Fractures in Athletes

Type	Treatment
• Type I (nondisplaced)	Minimal immobilization and early motion
• Type II	ORIF* and early motion
• Type III	ORIF and early motion if possible
• Type IV (comminuted)	Radial head resection; check distal joint (Essex-Lopresti injury); guarded prognosis for return to sports

*Open reduction and internal fixation

REHABILITATION PROTOCOL

Radial Head Fracture

Type I fracture or type II or III fracture treated with ORIF.

Phase 1—Immediate Motion Phase

- Goals:
  Decrease pain and inflammation.
  Regain full wrist and elbow ROM.
  Retard muscular atrophy.

1 week
- Begin elbow active ROM and active-assisted ROM; minimal accepted ROM (15 to 105 degrees) by 2 weeks.
- Begin putty/gripping exercises.
- Begin isometric strengthening exercises (elbow and wrist).
- Begin isotonic strengthening exercises for wrist.

Phase 2—Intermediate Phase

- Goals:
  Maintain full elbow ROM.
  Progress elbow strengthening exercises.
  Gradually increase functional demands.

3 weeks
- Initiate shoulder strengthening exercises; concentrate on rotator cuff.
- Continue ROM exercises for elbow (full flexion/extension).
- Initiate light resistance elbow flexion/extension (1 lb).
- Initiate active-assisted ROM and passive ROM supination/pronation to tolerance.
  Continued

REHABILITATION PROTOCOL—cont'd

Radial Head Fracture

Phase 2—Intermediate Phase—cont'd

6 weeks
- Continue active-assisted ROM and passive ROM supination/pronation to full range.
- Progress shoulder program.
- Progress elbow strengthening exercises.

Phase 3—Advanced Strengthening Phase
- Goals:
  Maintain full elbow ROM.

Increase strength, power, endurance. Gradually initiate sporting activities.

7 weeks
- Continue active-assisted ROM and passive ROM to full supination/pronation.
- Initiate eccentric elbow flexion/extension.
- Initiate plyometric exercise program.
- Continue isotonic program forearm, wrist, and shoulder.
- Continue until 12 weeks.

Elbow Arthroplasty

Contraindications to elbow arthroplasty include the following:
- Active infection.
- Absent flexors or flail elbow from motor paralysis.
- Noncompliant patient with respect to activity limitations.
- Inadequate posterior skin quality.
- Inadequate bone stock or ligamentous instability with resurfacing implants.
- Neurotrophic joint.

Elbow prostheses are classified as semiconstrained (loose-hinge or sloppy-hinge), nonconstrained (minimally constrained), or fully constrained. Fully constrained prostheses are no longer used because of their unacceptable failure rate.

REHABILITATION PROTOCOL

Total Elbow Replacement*

3 days
- Remove bulky dressing and replace with light compressive dressing.
- Begin active ROM exercises for the elbow and forearm 6 times a day for 10 to 15 minutes.

  ■ *Active ROM exercises should be performed with the elbow close to the body to avoid excessive stretch of the reconstructed elbow collateral ligaments.*
- Fit an elbow extension splint to be worn between exercise sessions and at night.

2 weeks
- Passive ROM exercises may be initiated to the elbow.
- Functional electrical stimulation (FES) may be initiated to stimulate biceps, triceps, or both.

6 weeks
- Discontinue elbow extension splint during the day if elbow stability is adequate.
- ROM exercises may now be performed with elbow away from body.

8 weeks
- Discontinue elbow extension splint at night.
- Initiate gradual, gentle strengthening exercises for hand and forearm. Light resistance may be begun to the elbow.
- Perform therapy within the patient's comfort level.

*From Cannon NM: *Diagnosis and treatment manual for physicians and therapists*, ed 3, 1991, The Hand Rehabilitation Center of Indiana, PC.

CHAPTER THREE

Rehabilitation of the Shoulder

FRANK W. JOBE, MD

DIANE MOYNE SCHWAB, PT

KEVIN E. WILK, PT

JAMES R. ANDREWS, MD

General Principles

The glenohumeral joint is inherently unstable, exhibiting the greatest amount of motion of any joint in the body. The humeral head is stabilized through a complex array of both static (passive) and dynamic (active) stabilizers. These mechanisms provide the necessary balance between functional mobility and stability.

The low success rate in returning these athletes to competition after surgical decompression reinforces the importance and desirability of both prevention of injury and nonoperative management.

Impingement Syndrome

PROGRESSIVE STAGES OF IMPINGEMENT

(See the box on p. 105.)

Neer demonstrated that the functional arc of the shoulder is forward, not lateral, and impingement occurs predominantly against the anterior edge of the acromion and the coracoacromial ligament.

■ *Both structural and functional factors may contribute to subacromial impingement.*

A common problem in overhead athletes (such as throwers, tennis players, and swimmers) is shoulder pain caused by impingement of the rotator cuff tendons underneath the coracoacromial arch.

■ *Shoulder impingement may be primary or secondary. Differentiating primary impingement from secondary impingement is crucial to proper management and rehabilitation. If secondary impingement is managed as "classic" impingement (repeated subacromial injections, acromioplasty), the underlying instability problem will not be adequately corrected.*

SECONDARY IMPINGEMENT

Secondary impingement is a relative decrease in the subacromial space caused by *instability* of the glenohumeral joint or by functional scapulothoracic instability. Secondary impingement caused by glenohumeral instability often is triggered by weakness of the rotator cuff mechanism and the biceps tendon, leading to overload of the passive restraints during throwing and resulting in glenohumeral laxity. The active restraints of the glenohumeral joint (the rotator cuff and biceps tendon) attempt to stabilize the humeral head; however, they eventually fatigue and weaken, with

Progressive Stages of Impingement

Stage 1: Edema and Inflammation

Typical age	Less than 25 years, but may occur at any age
Clinical course	Reversible lesion
Physical signs	• Tenderness to palpation over the greater tuberosity of the humerus
	• Tenderness along anterior ridge of acromion
	• Painful arc of abduction between 60 to 120 degrees, increased with resistance at 90 degrees
	• Positive impingement sign
	• Shoulder range of motion (ROM) may be restricted with significant subacromial inflammation

Stage 2: Fibrosis and Tendonitis

Typical age	25 to 40 years
Clinical course	Not reversible by modification of activity Stage 1 signs plus the following:
Physical signs	• Greater degree of soft tissue crepitus may be felt because of scarring in the subacromial space
	• Catching sensation with lowering of arm at approximately 100 degrees
	• Limitation of active and passive ROM

Stage 3: Bone Spurs and Tendon Ruptures

Typical age	Greater than 40 years
Clinical course	Not reversible
Physical signs	Stages 1 and 2 signs plus the following:
	• Limitation of ROM, more pronounced with active motion
	• Atrophy of infraspinatus
	• Weakness of shoulder abduction and external rotation
	• Biceps tendon involvement
	• Acromioclavicular joint tenderness

resultant abnormal translation of the humeral head and mechanical impingement of the rotator cuff by the coracoacromial arch.

In throwing athletes, secondary impingement may be caused by subacromial impingement due to functional scapular instability. Weakness of the scapulothoracic muscles leads to abnormal positioning of the scapula. Disruption of the scapulohumeral rhythm occurs, leading to impingement of the rotator cuff under the coracoacromial arch, because humeral elevation is not synchronized with scapular elevation and upward rotation. With this disruption, the acromion is not elevated sufficiently to allow unrestricted passage of the rotator cuff under the coracoacromial arch.

Because of these factors, rehabilitation should be directed at strengthening both the rotator cuff and the scapular rotators to establish proper scapulohumeral rhythm. Rotator cuff strengthening decreases impingement by improving humeral head depression and preventing excessive superior migration of the humeral head during arm elevation. Scapular rotator strengthening ensures that the scapula follows the humerus, providing dynamic stability and synchronization of the scapulohumeral rhythm.

PRIMARY IMPINGEMENT

Primary impingement is impingement of the rotator cuff beneath the coracoacromial arch. This is a *mechanical* impingement that may result from subacromial crowding.

■ *Instability of the glenohumeral joint is **absent** in primary impingement.*

IMPINGEMENT IN THE OVERHEAD ATHLETE

Overhead athletes usually exhibit adaptive changes in motion because of the repetitive stresses, and these adaptations often result in acquired laxity anteriorly and a loss of flexibility in the posterior muscles and posterior capsule. Because posterior capsular tightness often causes anterosuperior migration of the humeral head, contributing to impingement, posterior capsular stretching is useful (Fig. 3-1).

■ *Anterior capsular stretching should be avoided or carefully evaluated to prevent exacerbation of preexisting anterior capsular instability.*

Biomechanics of Throwing

The overhead throwing motion has been divided into six stages (Fig. 3-2).

Pain in the late cocking phase can be felt *anteriorly* and *superiorly* secondary to anterior subluxation of the humerus, with aggravated impingement of the rotator cuff as the humeral head moves superiorly. In the late cocking and early acceleration phases, initial symptoms may be posterior, probably secondary to posterior capsular and rotator cuff strain as the glenohumeral joint attempts to balance the occult anterior laxity.

A 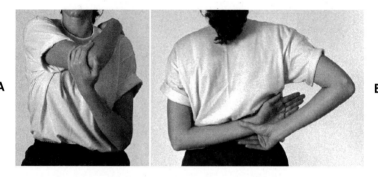 B

Figure 3-1 **A,** Crossed-arm adduction for posterior capsular stretching. **B,** The posterior capsule should be stretched to achieve full internal rotation.

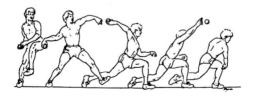

Figure 3-2 Five stages of the overhand throwing motion: stage 1, windup; stage 2, early cocking; stage 3, late cocking; stage 4, acceleration; and stage 5, follow-through. (From Glousman RE et al: Dynamic EMG analysis of the throwing shoulder with glenohumeral instability, *J Bone Joint Surg* 70A:220, 1988.)

General Rehabilitation Principles in Throwing Athletes (Hawkins and Litchfield)

Functional Plane of Motion

Rehabilitation of the shoulder should be performed in functional planes of motion. Most exercises are done anterior to the scapular plane or in the scapular plane. This generally is a pain-free range. Exercises in the coronal plane should be avoided because this is a nonfunctional motion and often exacerbates impingement.

Short Lever Arm

Early in the rehabilitation program, especially in athletes with pain, passive and active movements should be initiated with the elbow flexed to decrease torque around the shoulder. During the resisted and strengthening phases of rehabilitation, loads should be applied with the arms close to the body and the elbows flexed to shorten the lever arm. Electromyogram (EMG) analysis has documented high levels of supra-spinatus activity with straight-arm resisted exercises in scapular-plane rehabilitation. This long lever arm often induces pain and should be avoided by bending the elbow of the athlete with painful shoulders.

Deceleration Musculature

Conditioning and eccentric strengthening should be included for the muscles prominent in the deceleration phase of throwing (i.e., latissimus dorsi, biceps brachii). The shoulder encounters enormous stresses in this phase.

Scapular Platform

A stable scapular platform and synchronization of the scapulohumeral rhythm are important in any rehabilitation or conditioning program.

Stretching

Most overhead athletes have limited internal rotation, a tight posterior capsule, and excessive external rotation. Historically, shoulder stretching has been done in many directions; however, stretching of the anterior capsule and exacerbation of underlying anterior subluxation or instability is unwise. Increasing internal rotation and eliminating posterior capsular tightness have been shown to increase the athlete's performance. A rigorous posterior capsular stretching program is indicated. (See Fig. 3-1.)

Progression of Exercise Program

The rehabilitation program should gradually increase forces and loading rates in a manner that reproduces the athlete's specific functional demands.

Rotator Cuff Tendonitis and Tears in Throwing Athletes

In throwing athletes, rotator cuff tendonitis may be caused by mechanical abrasion, overuse, excessive anterior translation of the humeral head within the glenohumeral joint space, or a combination of these factors. Considerations in the choice of a rehabilitation protocol include (1) the degree of shoulder stability, (2) the duration of the condition (acute or chronic), (3) the strength and endurance of the shoulder girdle musculature, (4) the performance requirements of the athlete's sport, and (5) the flexibility of the soft tissues around the shoulder. (See *Clinical Orthopaedic Rehabilitation* for rotator cuff tendonitis rehabilitation. See p. 110 for rotator cuff tear rehabilitation.)

REHABILITATION PROTOCOL

Repair (Deltoid Splitting) of Type I Rotator Cuff Injury (Small Tear [Less Than 1 cm]) WILK AND ANDREWS

Phase 1—Protective Phase (week 0 to 6)

GOALS
- Gradual return to full ROM
- Increase shoulder strength
- Decrease pain

0 to 3 weeks
- Fit sling for comfort (1 to 2 weeks).
- Perform pendulum exercises.
- Initiate active-assisted ROM exercises (L-bar exercise).
  Employ ROM exercises in a nonpainful range, with a gentle and gradual increase of motion to tolerance.
- Use rope and pulley for flexion (only).
- Perform elbow ROM, hand gripping.
- Begin isometrics (submaximal, subpainful isometrics):

  Abductors
  External rotators
  Internal rotators
  Elbow flexors
  Shoulder flexors
- Use pain-control modalities (ice, high-voltage galvanic stimulation [HVGS]).

3 to 6 weeks
- Progress all exercises (continue all above exercises).
- Perform active-assisted ROM L-bar exercises ER/IR (shoulder at 45 degrees abduction).
- Begin surgical tubing ER/IR (arm at side).
- Initiate humeral head stabilization exercises.

Phase 2—Intermediate Phase (7 to 12 weeks)

GOALS
- Full, nonpainful ROM
- Improve strength and power
- Increase functional activities; decrease residual pain

7 to 10 weeks
- Perform active-assisted ROM exercises (L-bar):

  Flexion to 170 to 180 degrees

  Perform ER/IR at 90 degrees abduction of shoulder:

  ER to 75 to 90 degrees

  IR to 75 to 85 degrees

- Perform ER exercises with 0 degrees abduction:

  ER to 30 to 40 degrees

- Perform strengthening exercises for shoulder.
- Perform exercise tubing ER/IR with arm at side.

  Use isotonics dumbbell exercises for the following:

  Deltoid

  Supraspinatus

  Elbow flexors

  Scapular muscles

- Use upper body ergometer.
- Full ROM is the goal of weeks 8 to 10.

10 to 12 weeks
- Continue all above exercises.
- Initiate isokinetic strengthening (scapular plane).
- Initiate side-lying ER/IR exercises (dumbbell).
- Initiate neuromuscular scapulae control exercises.

Phase 3—Advanced Strengthening Phase (weeks 13 to 21)

GOALS
- Maintain full, nonpainful ROM
- Improve shoulder complex strength
- Improve neuromuscular control
- Gradual return to functional activities.

13 to 18 weeks
- Begin active stretching program for the shoulder.

  Use active-assisted ROM L-bar flexion, ER/IR.

  Continued

REHABILITATION PROTOCOL—cont'd

Repair (Deltoid Splitting) of Type I Rotator Cuff Injury (Small Tear [Less Than 1 cm])   WILK AND ANDREWS

Phase 3—Advanced Strengthening Phase (weeks 13 to 21)—cont'd

13 to 18 weeks —cont'd
- Perform capsular stretches.
- Initiate aggressive strengthening program (isotonic program):
  - Shoulder flexion
  - Shoulder abduction
  - Supraspinatus
  - ER/IR
  - Elbow flexors/extensors
  - Scapular muscles
- Perform an isokinetic test (modified neutral position) at week 14:
  - ER/IR at 180 and 300 degrees per second
- Begin general conditioning program.

18 to 21 weeks
- Continue all exercises listed above.
- Initiate interval sport program.

Phase 4—Return to Activity Phase (21 to 26 weeks)
GOALS
- Gradual return to recreational sport activities

21 to 26 weeks
- Perform isokinetic test (modified neutral position).
- Continue to comply to interval sport program.
- Continue basic ten exercises (p. 128) for strengthening and flexibility.

REHABILITATION PROTOCOL

Repair (Deltoid Splitting) of Type II Rotator Cuff Injury (Medium to Large Tear [Greater Than 1 cm and Less Than 5 cm]) WILK AND ANDREWS

Phase 1—Protective Phase (0 to 6 weeks)

GOALS
- Gradual increase in ROM
- Increase shoulder strength
- Decrease pain and inflammation

0 to 3 weeks
- Fit brace or sling (physician determines).
- Begin pendulum exercises.
- Perform active-assisted ROM exercises (L-bar exercise):
  Flexion to 125 degrees
  ER/IR (shoulder at 40 degrees abduction) to 30 degrees
- Perform passive ROM to tolerance.
- Use rope and pulley—flexion.
- Perform elbow ROM and hand-gripping exercises.

- Begin submaximal isometrics:
  Flexors
  Abductors
  ER/IR
  Elbow flexors
- Use ice and pain modalities.

3 to 6 weeks
- Discontinue brace or sling.
- Continue all exercises listed above.
- Perform active-assisted ROM exercises:
  Flexion to 145 degrees
  ER/IR (performed at 65 degrees abduction) range to tolerance

Continued

Repair (Deltoid Splitting) of Type II Rotator Cuff Injury (Medium to Large Tear [Greater Than 1 cm and Less Than 5 cm])   WILK AND ANDREWS

Phase 2—Intermediate Phase (7 to 14 weeks)
GOALS
- Full, nonpainful ROM (10 weeks)
- Gradual increase in strength
- Decrease pain

7 to 10 weeks	• Perform active-assisted ROM L-bar exercises: Flexion to 160 degrees ER/IR (performed at 90 degrees shoulder abduction) to tolerance (greater than 45 degrees) • Perform strengthening exercises: Use exercise tubing ER/IR, arm at side. Initiate humeral head stabilizing exercise. Initiate dumbbell strengthening exercises for the following:	Deltoid Supraspinatus Elbow flexion/extension Scapular muscles
10 to 14 weeks		• Continue all exercises listed above (full ROM by 10 to 12 weeks). • Begin isokinetic strengthening (scapular plane). • Begin side-lying ER/IR exercises (dumbbell). • Begin neuromuscular control exercises for scapular. NOTE: Patient must be able to elevate arm without shoulder and scapular hiking before initiating isotonics; if unable, maintain on humeral head stabilizing exercises.

Phase 3—Advanced Strengthening Phase (15 to 26 weeks)

GOALS
- Maintain full, nonpainful ROM
- Improve strength of shoulder
- Improve neuromuscular control
- Gradual return to functional activities

15 to 20 weeks
- Continue active-assisted ROM exercise with L-bar:
  Flexion, ER, IR
- Perform self-capsular stretches.
- Begin aggressive strengthening program:
  Shoulder flexion
  Shoulder abduction (to 90 degrees)
  Supraspinatus
  ER/IR
  Elbow flexors/extensors
  Scapular muscles
- Begin conditioning program.

21 to 26 weeks
- Continue all exercises listed above.
- Use isokinetic test (modified neutral position) for ER/IR at 180 and 300 degrees per second.
- Begin interval sport program.

Phase 4—Return to Activity Phase (24 to 28 weeks)

GOALS
- Gradual return to recreational sport activities

24 to 28 weeks
- Continue all strengthening exercises.
- Continue all flexibility exercises.
- Continue progression on interval programs.

REHABILITATION PROTOCOL

Repair (Deltoid Splitting) of Type III Rotator Cuff Injury (Large to Massive Tear [Greater Than 5 cm])   WILK AND ANDREWS

Phase 1—Protective Phase (0 to 8 weeks)

0 to 4 weeks	• Fit brace or sling (determined by physician).
	• Begin pendulum exercises.
	• Perform passive ROM to tolerance:
	  Flexion
	  ER/IR (shoulder at 45 degrees abduction)
	• Perform elbow ROM.
	• Perform hand gripping exercises.
	• Initiate continuous passive motion (CPM).
	• Use submaximal isometrics:
	  Abductors
	  ER/IR
	  Elbow flexors
	• Use ice and pain modalities.
	• Perform gentle active-assisted ROM with L-bar at 2 weeks.

4 to 8 weeks	• Discontinue brace or sling.
	• Perform active-assisted ROM with L-bar:
	  Flexion to 100 degrees
	  ER/IR (shoulder 45 degrees abduction) 40 degrees
	• Continue pain modalities.

Phase 2—Intermediate Phase (8 to 14 weeks)

GOALS	• Establish full ROM (12 weeks) • Gradually increase strength • Decrease pain

8 to 10 weeks	• Perform active-assisted ROM L-bar exercises:
	  Flexion to tolerance
	  ER/IR (shoulder 90 degrees abduction) to tolerance

Phase 2—Intermediate Phase (8 to 14 weeks)—cont'd

8 to 10 weeks —cont'd
- Begin isotonic strengthening:
  Deltoid to 90 degrees
  ER/IR side-lying
  Supraspinatus
  Biceps/triceps
  Scapular muscles
  Flexion, ER, IR
- Perform self-capsular stretches.
- Begin aggressive strengthening program:
  Shoulder flexion
  Shoulder abduction (to 90 degrees)
  Supraspinatus
  ER/IR
  Elbow flexors/extensors
  Scapular strengthening
- Begin conditioning program.

10 to 14 weeks
- Continue all exercises listed above (full ROM by 12 to 14 weeks).
- Begin neuromuscular control exercises.
  If patient is unable to elevate arm without shoulder hiking (scapulothoracic substitution), maintain on humeral head stabilizing exercises.

Phase 3—Advanced Strengthening Phase (15 to 26 weeks)

GOALS
- Maintain full, nonpainful ROM
- Improve strength of shoulder
- Improve neuromuscular control
- Gradual return to functional activities

15 to 20 weeks
- Continue active-assisted ROM exercise with L-bar:

21 to 26 weeks
- Continue all exercises listed above.
- Use isokinetic test (modified neutral position) for ER/IR at 180 and 300 degrees per second.
- Begin interval sport program.

Phase 4—Return to Activity Phase (24 to 28 weeks)

GOAL
- Gradual return to recreational sport activities

24 to 28 weeks
- Continue all strengthening exercises.
- Continue all flexibility exercises.
- Continue progression on interval program.

REHABILITATION PROTOCOL

Arthroscopic Subacromial Decompression—Intact Rotator Cuff
WILK AND ANDREWS

This evaluation-based rehabilitation protocol is used for patients who have a stable shoulder (intact rotator cuff) after arthroscopic shoulder decompression (Fig. 3-3).

Phase 1—Immediate Motion Phase (Days 1 to 14)
GOALS
- Prevent negative effects of immobilization
- Regain full, pain-free ROM
- Retard muscular atrophy
- Reduce pain and inflammation

- Begin pendulum exercises to promote early motion and minimize pain.
- Begin active-assisted exercises with T-bar:
  Shoulder flexion
  Shoulder extension

  IR and ER
  Begin rotation exercises at 0 degrees of abduction; progress to 45 degrees of abduction, eventually gaining 90 degrees of abduction.
  Carefully monitor progression.
- Begin capsular stretching for anterior, posterior, and inferior capsule, using opposite arm and hand to create overpressure.
- Use modalities to control pain and inflammation:
  Ice
  HVGS
  Ultrasound
  Nonsteroidal antiinflammatory drugs (NSAIDs)

When	Immediate Motion Phase 7-14 days	Intermediate Phase 2-6 weeks	Dynamic Strengthening Phase 6-12 weeks	Return To Activity 12-16 weeks
Criteria for progression	• Stable Shoulder	• Minimal pain • Nearly complete ROM • Strength at least 4/5 (good)	• Painless full ROM • No pain • Strength 70% of contralateral side • No impingement by exam	• Full painless ROM • No pain • Muscle strength that fulfills criteria for sport (isometric/isokinetic) • Satisfactory PE
Signs	• Inflammation • Pain • Loss of ROM • Weakness	• Pain • ROM • Weakness • Poor neuromuscular control		• Isokinetic dynamometer 85% contralateral side

Rx	• Passive & active assisted motion exercises
	  -pendulum
	  -T-bar
	• Capsular stretches
	• Strengthening
	  -submaximal
	  -isometrics
	• Modalities
	  -ice
	  -high voltage galvanic stim
	• NSAIDS
		• Active assisted ROM
		• Active ROM
		• Aggressive stretching
		• Strengthening
		  -isotonic dumbbell
		  -submaximal
		  -isokinetics
		• Neuromuscular control exercises
		  -PNF
		• Cardiovascular fitness
			• Aggressive stretching
			• Strengthening
			  -constant loading (eccentric & concentric)
			  -isokinetics
			  -manual resistance
			  -plyometrics
			• Neuromuscular control exercises
				• Interval program

Goals	• Prevent effects of immobilization • Full, painless ROM • Prevent atrophy • Reduce pain & inflammation	• Normalize full ROM • Regain & improve strength • Improve neuromuscular control • Eliminate pain & inflammation	• Improve strength, power, endurance • Improve neuromuscular control • Prepare for gradual return to functional activities	• Unrestricted activity • Maintain normal motion & function

Figure 3-3 Evaluation-based rehabilitation protocol: rehabilitation after arthroscopic shoulder decompression. The protocol is based on four phases: 1, immediate motion phase of 7 to 14 days; 2, intermediate phase of 2 to 6 weeks; 3, dynamic strengthening phase of 6 to 12 weeks; and 4, return to activity phase of 12 to 16 weeks. (From Wilk KE, Andrews JR: *Orthopedics* 16(3):349, 1993.)

Continued

REHABILITATION PROTOCOL—cont'd

Arthroscopic Subacromial Decompression—Intact Rotator Cuff
WILK AND ANDREWS

Phase 2—Intermediate Phase (2 to 6 weeks)

CRITERIA FOR PROGRESSION TO PHASE 2
- Minimal pain and tenderness
- Nearly complete motion
- Good (⅘) strength

GOALS
- Normalize full, pain-free motion and shoulder arthrokinematics
- Improve muscular strength
- Improve neuromuscular control
- Eliminate residual inflammation and pain

- Continue active-assisted exercises with more aggressive stretching at all end ranges.
- Use joint mobilization techniques for capsular restriction, especially the posterior capsule.

- *Posterior capsular tightness causes superior and anterior humeral head elevation during shoulder elevation, contributing to impingement. Emphasize stretching of this portion of the capsule.*
- Begin strengthening: progress from isometric to isotonic dumbbell exercises:
  Shoulder abduction to 90 degrees
  Supraspinatus (scaption: empty can) (Fig. 3-4)
  Shoulder flexion to 90 degrees
  Side-lying IR and ER (Fig. 3-5)
  Elbow flexion and extension

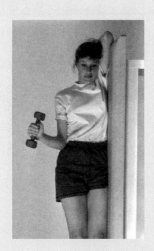

Figure 3-5 External rotation strengthening with weights.

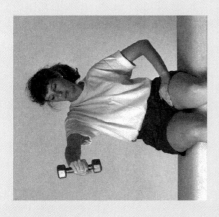

Figure 3-4 Isotonic resistance exercise for the supraspinatus muscle (scaption).

Continued

REHABILITATION PROTOCOL—cont'd

Arthroscopic Subacromial Decompression—Intact Rotator Cuff
WILK AND ANDREWS

Phase 2—Intermediate Phase (2 to 6 weeks)—cont'd
GOALS—cont'd

- Perform scapular stabilizing exercises: emphasize scapular movements through manual resistance during neuromuscular control exercises:

  Scapular retraction (rhomboideus, middle trapezius)

  Scapular protraction (serratus anterior)

  Scapular depression (latissimus dorsi, trapezius, serratus anterior)

- Begin submaximal isokinetics in the plane of the scapula or in the modified neutral position late in this phase.

■ *Rathburn and Macnab have shown that with the arm adducted (at the side), a zone of avascularity exists in the supraspinatus. With abduction, vascularity improves. Thus, Wilk and Andrews recommend that rotator cuff exercises be performed with the arm slightly abducted.*

- Begin proprioceptive neuromuscular facilitation exercises in the D_2 flexion/extension pattern with isometric holds (rhythmic stabilization).

Phase 3—Dynamic Strengthening (6 to 12 weeks)

CRITERIA FOR PROGRESSION TO PHASE 3
- Full, painless ROM
- No pain or tenderness
- 70% strength of contralateral shoulder
- Stable shoulder on clinical exam (negative impingement)

STRENGTHENING
- Begin fundamental shoulder exercises (see the boxes) to ensure progressive improvement in shoulder strength. These exercises are chosen because of the observed high EMG activity of the shoulder and scapulothoracic musculature.
- Progress isokinetics, manual resistive, and eccentric exercises.
- For competitive athletes who require enhanced strength and who are exposed to large deceleration stresses, begin a plyometric program:
  Plyometric drills with eccentric loading phase before concentric response phase
  Plyoball, exercise tubing, and/or wall (Fig. 3-6)
  Continued

GOALS
- Improve shoulder complex strength, power, endurance
- Improve neuromuscular control and shoulder proprioception
- Prepare for gradual return to functional activities

WARNING SIGNALS
- Loss of motion (especially IR)
- Lack of strength progression (especially abductors)
- Continued pain (especially night pain)

REHABILITATION PROTOCOL—cont'd

Arthroscopic Subacromial Decompression—Intact Rotator Cuff
WILK AND ANDREWS

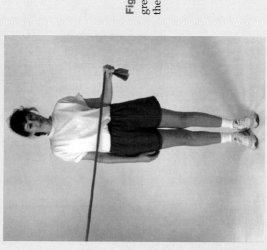

Figure 3-6 With the elbow close to the body and flexed 90 degrees, the shoulder is externally rotated against the resistance of the band.

Phase 4—Return to Activity (12 to 16 weeks)

CRITERIA FOR PROGRESSION TO PHASE 4	• Full, painless ROM • No pain or tenderness • Muscular strength (isokinetic/isometric) that fulfills established criteria • Satisfactory clinical exam	• Begin interval program (see box on p. 126): Throwing athletes, tennis and golf athletes Progressive, systematic interval program before returning to demands of sport For throwing athletes, monitor the number of throws, distance, intensity, and types of throws, and progress to enhance a return to competition.
GOALS	• Progressive return to unrestricted activity • Maintenance of normal shoulder strength and motion • Continue fundamental shoulder exercises (p. 128).	

Continued

Interval Throwing Program Following Arthroscopic Subacromial Decompression

45-Foot Phase

Step 1:
- A) Warm-up throwing
- B) 45 feet (25 throws)
- C) Rest 15 minutes
- D) Warm-up throwing
- E) 45 feet (25 throws)

Step 2:
- A) Warm-up throwing
- B) 45 feet (25 throws)
- C) Rest 10 minutes
- D) Warm-up throwing
- E) 45 feet (25 throws)
- F) Rest 10 minutes
- G) Warm-up throwing
- H) 45 feet (25 throws)

60-Foot Phase

Step 3:
- A) Warm-up throwing
- B) 60 feet (25 throws)
- C) Rest 15 minutes
- D) Warm-up throwing
- E) 60 feet (25 throws)

60-Foot Phase—cont'd

Step 4:
- A) Warm-up throwing
- B) 60 feet (25 throws)
- C) Rest 10 minutes
- D) Warm-up throwing
- E) 60 feet (25 throws)
- F) Rest 10 minutes
- G) Warm-up throwing
- H) 60 feet (25 throws)

90-Foot Phase

Step 5:
- A) Warm-up throwing
- B) 90 feet (25 throws)
- C) Rest 15 minutes
- D) Warm-up throwing
- E) 90 feet (25 throws)

Step 6:
- A) Warm-up throwing
- B) 90 feet (25 throws)
- C) Rest 10 minutes
- D) Warm-up throwing
- E) 90 feet (25 throws)

90-Foot Phase—cont'd

- F) Rest 10 minutes
- G) Warm-up throwing
- H) 90 feet (25 throws)

120-Foot Phase

Step 7:
- A) Warm-up throwing
- B) 120 feet (25 throws)
- C) Rest 15 minutes
- D) Warm-up throwing
- E) 120 feet (25 throws)

Step 8:
- A) Warm-up throwing
- B) 120 feet (25 throws)
- C) Rest 10 minutes
- D) Warm-up throwing
- E) 120 feet (25 throws)
- F) Rest 10 minutes
- G) Warm-up throwing
- H) 120 feet (25 throws)

150-Foot Phase

Step 9:
A) Warm-up throwing
B) 150 feet (25 throws)
C) Rest 15 minutes
D) Warm-up throwing
E) 150 feet (25 throws)

Step 10:
A) Warm-up throwing
B) 150 feet (25 throws)
C) Rest 10 minutes
D) Warm-up throwing
E) 150 feet (25 throws)
F) Rest 10 minutes
G) Warm-up throwing
H) 150 feet (25 throws)

180-Foot Phase

Step 11:
A) Warm-up throwing
B) 180 feet (25 throws)
C) Rest 15 minutes
D) Warm-up throwing
E) 180 feet (25 throws)

Step 12:
A) Warm-up throwing
B) 180 feet (25 throws)
C) Rest 10 minutes
D) Warm-up throwing
E) 180 feet (25 throws)
F) Rest 10 minutes
G) Warm-up throwing
H) 180 feet (25 throws)

180-Foot Phase—cont'd

Step 13:
A) Warm-up throwing
B) 180 feet (25 throws)
C) Rest 10 minutes
D) Warm-up throwing
E) 180 feet (25 throws)
F) Rest 10 minutes
G) Warm-up throwing
H) 180 feet (50 throws)

Step 14:
Begin throwing off the mound or return to respective position.

From Wilk RE, Andrews JR: Rehabilitation following arthroscopic subacromial decompression, *Orthopedics* 16(3):349, 1993.

Continued

REHABILITATION PROTOCOL—cont'd

Arthroscopic Subacromial Decompression—Intact Rotator Cuff
WILK AND ANDREWS

Fundamental Shoulder Exercises ("Basic Ten")

1. Rope and pulley flexion
2. L-bar flexion stretches
3. L-bar external rotation stretches
4. L-bar internal rotation stretches
5. External/internal rotation strengthening
6. Lateral raises to 90 degrees
7. Empty can
8. Passive ROM—horizontal abduction
9. Biceps curls
10. Self-capsular stretches

Throwers' Ten Program

1. Diagonal pattern D_2 extension and flexion
2. External/internal rotation at 0 degrees abduction
3. Shoulder abduction (palm down) to 90 degrees
4. Scaption with internal rotation
5. Prone horizontal abduction (neutral rotation); prone horizontal abduction (full external rotation, 100 degrees abduction)
6. Press-ups
7. Prone rowing
8. Push-ups
9. Elbow flexion/extension
10. Wrist flexion/extension; supination/pronation

Modified from Wilk KE et al: *Preventive and rehabilitative exercises for the shoulder and elbow*, ed 3, Birmingham, 1993, American Sports Medicine Institute.

Shoulder Instability

Shoulder instability may be based on several factors, including the direction and degree of the instability, as well as the time of onset and the frequency of dislocation.

TRAUMATIC ANTERIOR SHOULDER INSTABILITY

The most common cause of instability in the shoulder is traumatic anterior dislocation of the shoulder. The shoulder dislocates because it is forced into abduction and external rotation, overcoming the capsular labral restraints.

Individuals who sustain an initial dislocation before the age of 20 years as a result of minimal trauma have the highest risk of recurrent dislocation. Rowe and Sakellarides reported a 92% recurrence rate in individuals age 20 years or younger at the time of initial dislocation.

■ *Age at dislocation appears to be a more important factor than length of immobilization, specific rehabilitation program, or degree of initial trauma.*

Patients older than 40 years of age at initial dislocation probably should be immobilized for a briefer period than are younger patients, because the recurrence rate in this age group is low, and longer immobilization is more likely to lead to shoulder stiffness. Immobilization is continued only until pain subsides, typically in 7 to 10 days.

Although the essential pathologic lesion in younger patients (less than 25 years of age) may be disruption or stretching of the anterior capsule and ligamentous structures, weakening of the rotator cuff tendons is more common in patients more than 40 years of age. Rotator cuff tear should be suspected in patients older than 40 years, especially if persistent pain or weakness does not improve within 2 weeks of reduction.

For rehabilitation of arthroscopic anterior capsulolabral reconstruction in overhead athletes, please refer to *Clinical Orthopaedic Rehabilitation.*

REHABILITATION PROTOCOL

Acute Traumatic Anterior Shoulder Dislocation

- Immobilize young patients in a sling for 4 to 6 weeks. Patients older than 40 years are immobilized only until pain subsides.
- Begin active ROM exercises of elbow, wrist, and hand.
- Avoid positions of extreme adduction and ER during immobilization, as well as for 3 months after removal of sling.
- After immobilization is discontinued, gradually progress through rehabilitation program that emphasizes strengthening of the rotator cuff and scapular musculature (see the following protocol).

- Prerequisites for return to sports and overhead activities include full ROM, return of strength, and absence of pain.
- When the patient returns to athletic activities, a harness that limits abduction may be used to help avoid recurrent injury.
- If progress in therapy is slow, an arthrogram or magnetic resonance imaging (MRI) should be obtained to rule out a rotator cuff pathologic condition, especially in older patients.

REHABILITATION PROTOCOL

Anterior Capsular Shift Procedure: Regular WILK AND ANDREWS

The goal of this rehabilitation protocol is to return the patient/athlete to activity or sport as quickly and safely as possible, while maintaining a stable shoulder. The program is based on muscle physiology, biomechanics, anatomy, and the healing process following anterior capsular shift surgery, in which an incision is made into the ligamentous capsule of the shoulder, the capsule is pulled tighter, and is sutured together. The ultimate goal is a functional, stable shoulder and a pain-free return to the presurgery functional level.

Phase 1—Protection Phase (0 to 6 weeks)
GOALS   Allow healing of sutured capsule
           Begin early protected ROM
           Retard muscle atrophy
           Decrease pain and inflammation

0 to 2   • Precautions:
weeks   Sleep in immobilizer for 4 weeks

No overhead activities for 6 weeks
Wean from immobilizer and fit sling as soon as possible (determined by orthopaedist or therapists), approximately 3 to 4 weeks
• Begin gripping exercises with putty.
• Perform elbow flexion/extension and pronation/supination.
• Begin pendulum exercises (non-weighted).
• Perform rope and pulley active-assisted exercises:
    Shoulder flexion to 90 degrees
    Shoulder abduction to 60 degrees
• Perform T-bar exercises:
    ER to 15 to 20 degrees with arm abducted at 40 degrees
    Shoulder flexion/extension
• Perform active ROM, cervical spine.
                                    Continued

REHABILITATION PROTOCOL—cont'd

Anterior Capsular Shift Procedure: Regular   WILK AND ANDREWS

Phase 1—Protection Phase (0 to 6 weeks)—cont'd	
0 to 2 weeks— cont'd	• Begin isometrics: Flexors, extensors, ER, IR, abduction • Criteria for hospital discharge: Shoulder active-assisted ROM: flexion 90 degrees, abduction 45 degrees, ER 45 degrees Minimal pain and swelling "Good" proximal and distal muscle power
2 to 4 weeks	• Goals: Gradually increase ROM Normalize arthrokinematics Improve strength Decrease pain and inflammation • Perform ROM exercises: T-bar active-assisted exercises
2 to 4 weeks cont'd	ER to 25 degrees at 45 degrees shoulder abduction IR to 65 degrees at 45 degrees shoulder abduction Shoulder flexion/extension to tolerance Shoulder abduction to tolerance Shoulder horizontal abduction/adduction Rope and pulley flexion/extension *All* exercises are performed to tolerance; take to point of pain and/or resistance and hold. • Begin gentle self-capsular stretches. • Initiate gentle joint mobilization to reestablish normal arthrokinematics: Scapulothoracic joint Glenohumeral joint Sternoclavicular joint

Phase 1—Protection Phase (0 to 6 weeks)—cont'd

2 to 4 weeks—cont'd

- Perform strengthening exercises:
  Isometrics
  May begin tubing for ER/IR at 0 degrees
- Begin conditioning program for trunk, lower extremities, cardiovascular system.
- Use modalities, ice, and NSAIDs to decrease pain and inflammation.
- Increase strength
- Improve neuromuscular control

4 to 6 weeks

- Continue all exercises to tolerance.
- Perform ROM exercises:
  T-bar active-assisted exercises
  ER to 25 to 35 degrees at 45 degrees of shoulder abduction
  ER to 5 to 10 degrees at 90 degrees of shoulder abduction
  IR to 75 degrees at 90 degrees of shoulder abduction
  Continue all others to tolerance.

6 to 8 weeks

- Begin ROM exercises:
  T-bar active-assisted exercises at 90 degrees abduction
  Continue all exercises listed above.
  Gradually increase ROM to full ROM at week 12.
- Continue self-capsular stretches.
- Continue joint mobilization.
- Perform strengthening exercises:
  Begin isotonic dumbbell program:
  Side-lying ER
  Side-lying IR
  Shoulder abduction
  Supraspinatus
  Latissimus dorsi
  Rhomboids
  Biceps curl

Phase 2—Intermediate Phase (6 to 12 weeks)

GOALS

- Full, nonpainful ROM by 10 to 12 weeks
- Normalize arthrokinematics

REHABILITATION PROTOCOL—cont'd

Anterior Capsular Shift Procedure: Regular WILK AND ANDREWS

Phase 2—Intermediate Phase (6 to 12 weeks)—cont'd

6 to 8 weeks —cont'd
- Triceps curl
- Shoulder shrugs
- Push-ups into chair (serratus anterior)
- Continue tubing at 0 degrees for ER/IR.
- Begin neuromuscular control exercises for scapulothoracic joint.

8 to 10 weeks
- Continue all exercises.
- Begin tubing exercises for rhomboids, latissimus dorsi, biceps, and triceps.
- Begin aggressive stretching and joint mobilization if needed.

Phase 3—Dynamic Strengthening Phase (12 to 20 weeks)

12 to 17 weeks

GOALS:
- Improve strength, power, and endurance

CRITERIA TO ENTER PHASE 3
- Improve neuromuscular control
- Prepare athlete to begin throwing
- Full, nonpainful ROM (patient *must* fulfill this criteria)
- No pain or tenderness
- Strength 70% or more of contralateral side

EMPHASIS
- High-speed, high-energy strengthening exercises
- Eccentric exercises
- Diagonal patterns

12 weeks
- Perform throwers' ten program (p. 128).
- Perform tubing exercises:
  IR/ER at 0 degrees abduction (arm at side)
  Rhomboids
  Latissimus dorsi
  Biceps
  Diagonal patterns D_2 extension

Phase 3—Dynamic Strengthening Phase (12 to 20 weeks)—cont'd

12 weeks —cont'd
  Diagonal patterns
  - Perform dumbbell exercises for supraspinatus and deltoid.
  - Initiate serratus anterior strengthening (push-ups/floor).
  - Perform trunk, lower strengthening exercises.
  - Perform neuromuscular exercises.
  - Begin self-capsular stretches.

17 to 20 weeks
  - Continue all exercises.
  - Emphasize gradual return to recreational activities.

Phase 4—Return to Activity (20 to 28 weeks)

GOALS
  - Progressive increase in activities to prepare for full functional return
  - Full ROM
  - No pain or tenderness
  - Isokinetic test that fulfills criteria to throw
  - Satisfactory clinical exam

CRITERIA TO PROGRESS TO PHASE 4

20 to 24 weeks
  - Begin interval throwing programs (p. 126) if patient is a recreational athlete.
  - Continue tubing exercises (phase 3).
  - Continue ROM exercises.

REHABILITATION PROTOCOL

Anterior Capsulolabral Reconstruction (Open Procedure) in Throwing Athletes WILK AND ANDREWS

Phase 1—Immediate Motion Phase (0 to 7 weeks)

0 to 2 weeks	• Fit sling for comfort for 1 week.
	• Use immobilization brace for 4 weeks during sleep only.
	• Gentle active-assisted ROM exercises with T-bar:
	Flexion to tolerance (0 to 120 degrees)
	ER at 20 degrees abduction to tolerance (maximum 15 to 20 degrees)
	IR at 20 degrees abduction to tolerance (maximum 45 degrees)
	• Perform rope and pulley exercises.
	• Perform ROM exercises for hand and elbow.
	• Initiate isometrics (ER, IR, abduction, biceps).
	• Squeeze ball.
	• Perform elbow flexion/extension.
	• Use ice.
3 to 4 weeks	• Perform active-assisted ROM exercises with T-bar:
	Flexion to tolerance (maximum 120 to 140 degrees)
	ER at 45 degrees abduction (acceptable 20 to 30 degrees)
	IR at 45 degrees abduction (acceptable 45 to 60 degrees)
	• Begin light isotonics for shoulder musculature:
	Adduction
	Supraspinatus
	ER/IR
	Biceps
	• Begin scapular strengthening exercises:
	Rhomboids
	Trapezius
	Serratus anterior

Phase 1—Immediate Motion Phase (0 to 7 weeks)—cont'd

Weeks	
5 to 6 weeks	• Progress all active-assisted ROM with T-bar: Flexion (maximum 160 degrees) ER/IR at 90 degrees abduction ER to 45 to 60 degrees IR to 65 to 95 degrees • Upper body ergometer (UBE) arm at 90 degrees abduction. • Use diagonal patterns, manual resistance. • Progress all strengthening exercises.

Phase 2—Intermediate Phase (8 to 14 weeks)

Weeks	
8 to 10 weeks	• Progress to full ROM: Flexion to 180 degrees ER to 90 degrees IR to 85 degrees • Perform isokinetic strengthening exercises (neutral position). • Progress all strengthening exercises. • Perform scapular strengthening exercises.
10 to 14 weeks	• Continue all flexibility exercises, self-capsular stretches. • Begin throwers' ten program (p. 128) • UBE 90 degrees abduction. • Use diagonal pattern (manual resistance).

Phase 3—Advanced stage (4 to 6 months)

- Continue all flexibility exercises:
  ER/IR stretches
  Flexion stretch
  Self-capsular stretches
- Continue throwers' ten program.
- Perform isokinetics ER/IR (90/90 position).
- Use isokinetics test (throwers' series).
- Perform plyometric exercises.
- Begin interval throwing program (see rotator cuff section) if surgeon approves.

Phase 4—Return to Activity (6 to 9 months)

- Continue all strengthening exercises, including throwers' ten program.
- Continue all stretching exercises.

Prosthetic Shoulder Arthroplasty

Rehabilitation after shoulder arthroplasty depends on multiple factors, including the status of the soft tissues around the shoulder (intact or torn rotator cuff, size of tear, security of repair), the quality of the bone, the stability of the implant and the fixation technique used, any concomitant injuries or systemic illness, and the expectations of the patient.

Neer suggests dividing patients into two groups: (1) those who can participate in a reasonably *normal rehabilitation program* (such as patients with osteoarthritis), and (2) those with deficiencies of bone or muscle who must be placed in a *limited-goals rehabilitation program*. In the normal rehabilitation program, motion is begun early to prevent the formation of function-threatening adhesions or to retard their maturation. In the limited-goals group, rehabilitation is aimed at maintaining joint stability and obtaining a lesser ROM with reasonable muscle control. In this limited-goals setting, the initiation of exercises is delayed somewhat and the extent of passive or assisted early motion is reduced. Elevation usually is limited to 90 degrees and ER to 20 degrees. These limited arcs of movement allow more scar formation and greater joint mobility than in a more aggressive rehabilitation program.

REHABILITATION PROTOCOL

Shoulder Arthroplasty: Intact Rotator Cuff Rehabilitation
WILK AND ANDREWS

Phase 1—Immediate Motion Phase (0 to 4 weeks)

GOALS
- Increase passive ROM
- Decrease shoulder pain
- Retard muscular atrophy and prevent rotator cuff shutdown

EXERCISES
- Use CPM machine.
- Perform passive ROM exercises:
  Flexion (0 to 90 degrees)
  ER (at 30 degrees abduction) 0 to 30 degrees
  IR (at 30 degrees abduction) 0 to 35 degrees
- Perform pendulum exercises.
- Perform elbow and wrist ROM-exercises.
- Perform grasping exercises for hand.

- Use ice and modalities for pain control.
- Begin isometrics (ER, IR, abduction) on day 10.
- Use electrical muscle stimulation (if needed).
- Begin use of rope and pulley at week 2.
- Begin active-assisted ROM (ER, IR, flexion) with T-bar at week 2.

Phase 2—Active Motion Phase (4 to 10 weeks)

GOALS
- Improve shoulder strength
- Improve ROM
- Increase functional activities
- Decrease pain

Continued

REHABILITATION PROTOCOL—cont'd

Shoulder Arthroplasty: Intact Rotator Cuff Rehabilitation
WILK AND ANDREWS

Phase 2—Active Motion Phase (4 to 10 weeks)—cont'd

EXERCISES
- Use rope and pulley (flexion).
- Perform pendulum exercises.
- Perform active ROM (supine flexion).
- Perform seated flexion (short arc 45 to 90 degrees)
- Perform seated abduction.
- Begin exercise tubing ER/IR at 4 weeks.
- Use dumbbell for biceps/triceps.
- Practice scapulothoracic strengthening.
- Perform joint mobilization.

GOALS
- Strength (ER, IR, abduction) ⅗ of uninvolved extremity
- Improve strength of shoulder musculature
- Neuromuscular control of shoulder complex
- Improve functional activities
- Use exercise tubing: IR/ER.
- Practice dumbbell strengthening:
  Abduction
  Supraspinatus
  Scapulothoracic

EXERCISES
- Perform stretching exercises.
- Perform T-bar exercises.
- Perform rope and pulley exercises.

Phase 3—Strengthening Phase

CRITERIA FOR PROGRESSION TO PHASE 3
- Passive ROM: flexion 0 to 160 degrees
  ER 0 to 75 degrees
  IR 0 to 80 degrees

REHABILITATION PROTOCOL

Total Shoulder Arthroplasty: Tissue-Deficient Group WILK AND ANDREWS

The goal of the rehabilitation process is to provide greater joint stability to patients, while decreasing their pain and improving their functional status. The goal of the tissue-deficient group (bone loss, muscle loss) is joint stability and less joint mobility.

Phase 1—Immediate Motion Phase (0 to 4 weeks)

GOALS
- Increase passive ROM
- Decrease shoulder pain
- Retard muscular atrophy

EXERCISES
- Use CPM
- Perform passive ROM:
  Flexion 0 to 90 degrees
  ER (at 30 degrees abduction) 0 to 20 degrees
  IR (at 30 degrees abduction) 0 to 30 degrees
- Perform pendulum exercises.
- Perform ROM of elbow and wrist.
- Perform gripping exercises.

- Use isometrics:
  Abductors
  ER/IR
- Begin use of rope and pulley at 2 weeks.
- Perform active-assisted ROM exercises (when able).

Phase 2—Active Motion Phase (4 to 12 weeks)

GOALS
- Improve shoulder strength
- Improve ROM
- Decrease pain/inflammation
- Increase functional activities

EXERCISES
- Begin active-assisted ROM exercises with L-bar at 4 to 5 weeks or when tolerable:
  Flexion
  ER
  IR

Continued

REHABILITATION PROTOCOL—cont'd

Total Shoulder Arthroplasty: Tissue-Deficient Group   WILK AND ANDREWS

Phase 2—Active Motion Phase (4 to 12 weeks)—cont'd		IR of 45 to 55 degrees at 90 degrees abduction
EXERCISES— cont'd	• Continue use of rope and pulley (flexion).	
	• Continue pendulum exercises.	
	• Perform active ROM exercises:	
	Seated flexion (short arc 45 to 90 degrees)	
	Supine flexion (full available range)	
	Seated abduction (0 to 90 degrees)	
	Exercise tubing IR/ER (4 to 6 weeks)	
	Dumbbell biceps/triceps	
	Gentle joint mobilization (6 to 8 weeks)	
		GOALS • Strength level (ER, IR, abduction) ⅘ of involved extremity Note: *Some patients will never enter this phase.*
		• Improve strength of shoulder musculature
		• Improve and gradually increase functional activities
		• Continue exercise tubing (ER/IR).
		EXERCISES • Practice dumbbell strengthening: Abduction Supraspinatus Flexion
		• Perform stretching exercise.
		• Perform L-bar stretches: Flexion ER IR
Phase 3—Strengthening Phase		
CRITERIA FOR PROGRESSION TO PHASE 3	• Passive ROM: Flexion 0 to 120 degrees ER of 30 to 40 degrees at 90 degrees abduction	

Adhesive Capsulitis

For rehabilitation of adhesive capsulitis of the shoulder, please refer to *Clinical Orthopaedic Rehabilitation*.

Proximal Humeral Fractures

Codman described four segments of proximal humeral fractures: (1) the articular segment of the humeral head, (2) the greater tuberosity, (3) the lesser tuberosity, and (4) the humeral shaft. Neer classified fractures of the proximal humerus based on the identification of the four major fragments and their relationships to one other. When any of the four major segments is displaced more than 1 cm or angulated more than 45 degrees, the fracture is displaced. If no fragment is displaced, the fracture is a one-part fracture; 80% of proximal humeral fractures fall into this category. The primary concerns of this classification are the status of the blood supply of the humeral head and the relationship of the humeral head to the displaced parts and to the glenoid.

Bertoft et al. reported the greatest improvement in ROM after proximal humeral fractures occurred between 3 and 8 weeks after fracture. Return to normal function and motion may require 3 to 4 months. Bony healing is typically complete by 6 to 8 weeks in adults.

REHABILITATION PROTOCOL

Undisplaced Proximal Humeral Fractures   ROCKWOOD AND MATSEN

Rockwood and Matsen advocate a three-phase protocol devised by Neer.

Phase 1

1 day	• Begin hand, wrist, and elbow active ROM. • Support arm in a sling at the side or in a Velpeau position. • A swath may be needed in the immediate postfracture period for immobilization and comfort. • An axillary pad may be useful. • Periodic views in two perpendicular planes are essential to establish that the fracture is clinically stable and is not displacing.
7 to 10 days	• Begin gentle ROM exercises if clinical situation is stable. • Perform exercises 3 to 4 times a day for 20 to 30 minutes. • Applying hot packs 20 minutes before exercise may be beneficial. • Early in the program, an analgesic may be needed for pain control. • First begin pendulum exercises (Codman) with arm rotation in inward and outward circles. • Begin supine ER with a stick. Support the elbow and distal humerus with a folded towel or sheet to create a sense of security for the patient; 15 to 20 degrees of abduction may aid in performing these exercises.
3 to 5 weeks	• Begin assisted forward elevation. • Perform pulley exercises. • Perform ER with a stick. • Perform extension with a stick. • Perform isometric exercises.

Phase 2 (6 weeks to 2 months)

■ *Phase 2 exercises involve early active, resistive, and stretching exercises.*

- Begin supine active forward elevation as gravity is partially eliminated, thus making forward elevation easier.
- Progress forward elevation to an erect position with a stick in the unaffected hand to assist the involved arm in forward elevation.
- As strength is gained, may perform unassisted active elevation while erect, with emphasis on keeping the elbow bent and the arm close to the midline.
- Use Therabands of progressive strengths for internal rotators; external rotators; and anterior, middle, and posterior deltoid (3 sets of 10 to 15 repetitions at each exercise session).
- Perform stretching for forward elevation on the top of a door or wall, and stretching in the door jamb for ER.

- Raise arm over the head with the arms clasped.
- Perform ER and abduction of the arms with the hands placed behind the head.
- Help with IR by using the normal arm to pull the involved arm into IR.

Phase 3 (3 months)

- May use light weights after 3 months; start with 1 lb and increase in 1-lb increments with a 5-lb limit. If pain persists after using weights, eliminate or decrease weight.
- Replace Theraband with rubber tubing to increase resistance.
- Stretching on the end of the door and prone stretching for forward elevation are helpful.
- Perform functional activity for strength gain.

CHAPTER FOUR

Fractures of the Lower Extremity

THOMAS A. RUSSELL, MD
ANA K. PALMIERI, MD

Rehabilitation Rationale

The goals of successful treatment of lower extremity injuries are (1) restoration of functional range of motion (ROM) of all joints, (2) rehabilitation of all muscle-tendon units, and (3) unrestricted weight bearing. Rehabilitation of lower extremity injuries proceeds in stages based on the physiology of repair and the regeneration of the soft and hard tissues.

CLASSIFICATION

Two classification systems are used most often for soft tissue injuries: the *Tscherne* system for closed fractures and the *Gustilo and Anderson* system, with its later modification, for open fractures. Two other classification systems have been proposed more recently, the Mueller/AO classification and the Orthopaedic Trauma Association's modification of this classification, but these require time for validation and application to the literature.

The Tscherne classification serves primarily to alert the surgeon that significant crush and swelling of the soft tissue envelope may

---

TABLE 4-1 **The Tscherne Classification of Soft Tissue Injuries in Closed Fractures**

Grade 1   Soft tissue damage absent
Indirect forces
Torsion fractures

Grade 2   Superficial abrasion or contusion caused by fragment pressure from within
Mild-to-moderate fracture severity

Grade 3   Deep, contaminated abrasion associated with local skin or muscle contusion from direct trauma
Bumper injuries (pedestrian–motor vehicle)
Increased fracture severity with comminution or segmental injury

Grade 4   Skin extensively contused with crushed muscle
Muscle damage may be severe
Compartment syndromes common

TABLE 4-2 **The Gustilo-Anderson Classification of Soft Tissue Injury in Open Fractures**

Type I Wound less than 1 cm long
Minimal soft tissue damage, no signs of crush
Usually simple transverse or short oblique fracture with little comminution

Type II Wound more than 1 cm long
Slight-to-moderate crushing injury, no extensive soft tissue damage, flap, or avulsion
Moderate fracture comminution and contamination

Type III Extensive wound and soft tissue damage, including muscles, skin, and (often) neurovascular structures
Greater degree of fracture comminution and instability
High degree of contamination

IIIA Adequate soft tissue coverage of the fracture, despite extensive laceration, flaps, or high-energy trauma
This subtype includes highly comminuted or segmental fractures from high energy, regardless of the size of the wound. Type IIIA fractures do *not* require free flaps

IIIB Open fracture associated with extensive injury to or loss of soft tissue, with periosteal stripping and exposure of bone
Massive contamination and severe comminution
After debridement and irrigation, bone is exposed and requires a local flap or free flap

IIIC Any open fracture associated with an arterial injury that must be repaired, regardless of the extent of soft tissue injury
Open fractures with arterial injuries have projected amputation rates ranging from 25% to 90%

delay healing and lead to compartment syndromes or contractures (Table 4-1).

The Gustilo-Anderson classification of open fractures with subsequent modification helps to determine the relative risks of infection and nonunion (Table 4-2).

Open fractures generally are treated with repeat debridements until a stable soft tissue envelope is achieved by delayed primary closure or skin graft or flap coverage of the wound, preferably by 5 to 7 days. Stabilization of fractures with Gustilo-Anderson type I soft tissue injuries generally is the same as for closed fractures. Types II and III soft tissue injuries usually require stabilization of the fracture with intramedullary nailing or external fixation. Plate-and-screw fixation generally is reserved for displaced intraarticular fractures. Often the best treatment of severe type IIIC injuries is amputation, although the surgeon must obviously make this decision based on the clinical findings.

Acute bone grafting, sometimes used for **closed** fractures with bone loss from impaction, such as tibial plateau or pilon fractures, is not recommended for open fractures. At 6 to 12 weeks, bone grafting may be indicated in open fractures if the soft tissue envelope is stable and free of drainage, especially in fractures with bone loss. This situation is more common with open tibial fractures than with femoral fractures.

Occasionally *dynamization* is recommended to transfer stress from the implant to the extremity when external fixation systems or static interlocking intramedullary nails are used for fracture stabilization. Dynamization of static interlocking nails usually is an outpatient surgical procedure consisting of removal of the interlocking screws from the *longest fragment* of the injured bone. Nail dynamization usually is performed at 6 to 12 weeks in the tibia and at 12 to 24 weeks in the femur. Dynamization should not be performed with unstable fractures that would permit loss of alignment and significant leg-length inequality. These problems occur primarily in proximal and distal third fractures where the nail diameter and intramedullary canal diameter are mismatched, permitting translational and rotational instability after removal of the interlocking screw. Bone grafting as a biologic stimulus is typically used in these unstable fractures where dynamization is contraindicated.

GENERAL PRINCIPLES OF REHABILITATION

Rehabilitation after lower extremity fractures follows a general sequence of time-interval–dependent exercises and goals. Based on the relative average times of soft tissue and bony repair, the following four phases of rehabilitation are identified: **phase 1** (0 to 6 weeks), mobilization of adjacent joints and muscles and protected weight bearing for diaphyseal and metaphyseal fractures; **phase 2** (6 weeks to 3 months), strengthening and endurance exercises with progressive weight bearing; **phase 3** (3 to 6 months), progression to full unsupported weight bearing, agility and endurance-training, reentry into work and recreational activities; and **phase 4** (more than 6 months), resumption of normal activities.

A general outline of exercises and activities is shown in the box on pp. 152 and 153.

Exercises and Activities After Lower Extremity Fractures

Open-Chain Exercises

Characteristics

Distal segment is free

No weight bearing

Motion is only distal to axis of motion

Muscle contraction primarily concentric

Movements are usually isolated

Load is artificial

Velocity is predetermined

Stabilization is often artificial (straps and belts)

Usually in one cardinal plane of motion

Proprioceptive carry-over to functional activities questionable

Exercises often limited by equipment

Closed-Chain Exercises

Characteristics

Distal segment is not free

Partial weight bearing

Motion is both distal and proximal to the axis of motion

Muscle contraction includes concentric, eccentric, isometric, and isotonic

Movements are functional. Can emphasize one muscle group, but entire kinetic chain works together

Loads are physiological and through the entire kinetic chain

Variable velocity

Stabilization is a product of normal postural mechanisms

Motion takes place in all planes of joints

Significant proprioceptive carry-over to functional activities

Exercises limited only by imagination

Exercises

Isometrics
Straight leg raises
Knee ROM exercises
Terminal knee extension
Stationary bicycle
Proprioceptive neuromuscular facilitation (PNF)
Isokinetic exercise equipment
Weight equipment (in the seated position)

Exercises

Non–weight-bearing closed-chain exercises

Hip machine for uninvolved leg
Sitting with knee flexed, performing towel slides

Partial weight-bearing (PWB) closed-chain exercises

PWB minisquats
PWB wall sits
PWB lunges
Proprioception emphasis using BAPS board
Allow PWB ambulation when patient is 50% weight bearing

Full weight-bearing closed-chain exercises

Wall sits
Minisquats with or without resistance
Lunges
Proprioception with BAPS board or Fitter treadmill (retro walking and forward walking)
Pool
Stair machines (forward and reverse stance)
NordicTrack ski machines
Agility drills
Step-ups
Sliding lunges

Femoral Neck, Subtrochanteric, and Intertrochanteric Fractures

REHABILITATION RATIONALE

Femoral Neck Fractures

The most commonly used classification for femoral neck fractures is that of Garden, which is based on the amount of fracture displacement (Table 4-3).

For young patients with good bone stock in the femoral neck, head, and lateral shaft, femoral neck fractures can be treated with anatomic open reduction and, if required, internal fixation with three cancellous screws in a lag-screw fashion. In older patients with less structurally stable bone stock, a hip compression screw with an accessory screw or hemiarthroplasty may be more appropriate. Bipolar arthroplasty usually is recommended for patients with an expected life span of more than 5 years. For patients with less than 2 years expected life span who are household ambulators with insufficient bone quality for internal fixation, some type of hemiarthroplasty, such as the Austin Moore, probably is more appropriate.

General treatment considerations include the age and general health of the patient (Fig. 4-2).

TABLE 4-3 Garden Classification of Femoral Neck Fractures (Fig. 4-1)

Grade 1	Incomplete, impacted fracture
Grade 2	Nondisplaced fracture
Grade 3	Incompletely displaced fracture
Grade 4	Completely displaced fracture with no engagement of the two fragments

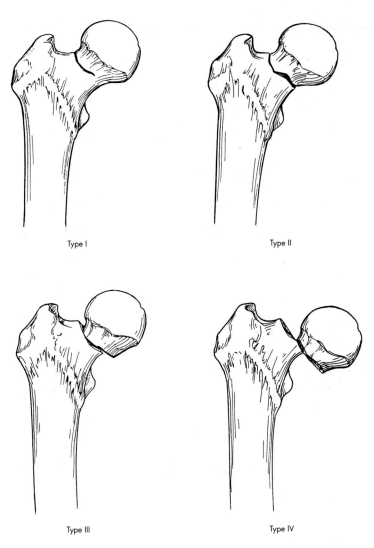

Type I

Type II

Type III

Type IV

Figure 4-1 Garden's classification. Treatment and avascular necrosis and union rates of femoral neck fractures are based on displacement. (From Kyle RF: *Fractures of the hip.* In Gustilo RB, Kyle RF, Templeman D, editors: *Fractures and dislocations,* St Louis, 1993, Mosby–Year Book.)

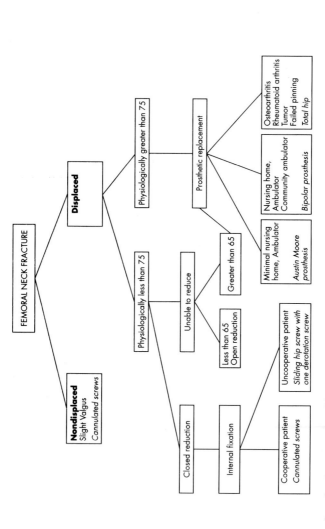

Figure 4-2 Flowchart for the treatment of femoral neck fractures. Treatment depends on the degree of displacement of the fracture and the age of the patient. Preexisting hip disease also dictates treatment. (From Kyle RF: *Fractures of the hip*. In Gustilo RB, Kyle RF, Templeman D, editors: *Fractures and dislocations*, St. Louis, 1993, Mosby–Year Book.)

Subtrochanteric Femoral Fractures

The key to stability of this fracture complex is very similar to that for intertrochanteric fracture: Is the medial column intact?

Russell and Taylor proposed a classification system (Fig. 4-3) that groups subtrochanteric fractures into four types to help determine the most appropriate type of operative stabilization. Fractures with stability of the lesser trochanter and an intact piriform fossa are similar to diaphyseal femoral fractures, and conventional interlocking nailing is advocated. In type IB fractures, the lesser trochanteric area and medial column are deficient, and there is no injury to the piriform fossa; for these fractures, a reconstruction-type intramedullary nail usually is recommended. In type IIA and IIB variants, the fracture extends from the subtrochanteric area up into the piriform fossa. If medial continuity is intact, as in type IA fractures, a standard hip compression screw can be used as for introchanteric fractures. Type IIB fractures, with comminution involving the piriformis fossa, medial comminution involving the lesser trochanter, and varying degrees of shaft comminution, frequently require indirect and open reduction techniques with hip compression screw fixation and autologous iliac bone grafting. If shaft comminution is extensive, occasionally open reduction and fixation with a reconstruction-type intramedullary nail are indicated because of the long diaphyseal fracture fragment.

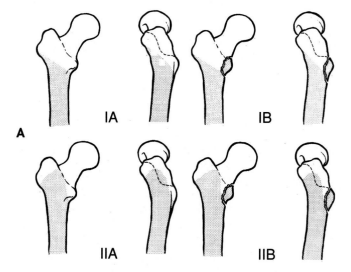

Figure 4-3 A, Russell-Taylor classification of subtrochantric fracture of femur based on involvement of piriformis fossa. Group 1 fractures do not extend into piriformis fossa: type IA—comminution and fracture lines extend from below lesser trochanter to femoral isthmus; type IB—fracture lines and comminution involve area of lesser trochanter to isthmus. Group 2 fractures extend proximally into greater trochanter and involve piriformis fossa: type IIA—without significant comminution or fracture of lesser trochanter; type IIB—with significant comminution of medial femoral cortex and loss of continuity of lesser trochanter. (From Russell TA: *Fractures of the hip and pelvis.* In Crenshaw AH, editor: *Campbell's operative orthopaedics,* ed 8, St. Louis, 1992, Mosby–Year Book.)

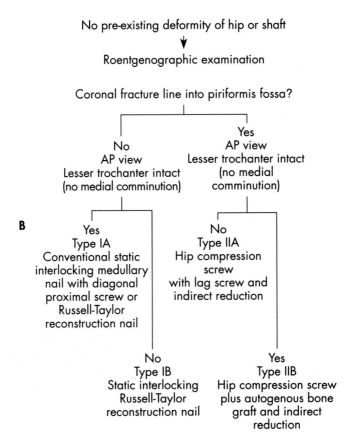

No pre-existing deformity of hip or shaft

Roentgenographic examination

Coronal fracture line into piriformis fossa?

	Yes
No	AP view
AP view	Lesser trochanter intact
Lesser trochanter intact	(no medial
(no medial comminution)	comminution)

B

Yes	No
Type IA	Type IIA
Conventional static	Hip compression
interlocking medullary	screw
nail with diagonal	with lag screw and
proximal screw or	indirect reduction
Russell-Taylor	
reconstruction nail	

No	Yes
Type IB	Type IIB
Static interlocking	Hip compression screw
Russell-Taylor	plus autogenous bone
reconstruction nail	graft and indirect
	reduction

Figure 4-3—cont'd B, Treatment algorithm for closed subtrochanteric femoral fractures based on the Russell-Taylor classification. (From Russell TA: *Fractures of hip and pelvis.* In Crenshaw AH: *Campbell's operative orthopaedics,* ed 8, St. Louis, 1992, Mosby–Year Book.

REHABILITATION PROTOCOL

Femoral Neck Fractures, Intertrochanteric Fractures, and Subtrochanteric Fractures

1 day

- Begin quadriceps sets, hamstring sets, gluteal sets, and ankle pumps.
- Perform gentle active-assisted abduction and adduction of the hip.
- Perform supine leg slides for flexion of the hip and knee.
- Institute bed mobility.
- Provide an exercise sheet for the patient and family. Explain and demonstrate each exercise; the patient then performs the exercises with assistance of the therapist.
- Provide occupational therapy to assist with ADLs.
- Perform upper extremity exercises, especially if the patient is to be bedridden for any period. The use of Therabands for independent exercises can be helpful, with PNF patterns performed by the therapist with appropriate resistance.

2 days

- Review the exercise sheet with the patient and family. Answer any questions and add new exercises to achieve a complete home program.
- Increase bed mobility (use of verbal cues more than assistance to get from supine to sitting will make the patient more independent).
- Increase ambulation with appropriate weight-bearing status (e.g. TDWB with walker, then PWB with walker, etc.).

3 to 7 days

- Encourage patient to be independent with exercises and assist in areas of difficulty.
- Perform straight leg raises in all directions, lying position and standing (if the patient has good balance).
- If the patient is weight bearing to tolerance, start weight-shifting exercises and minisquats.
- Begin gentle daily Thomas stretch of the anterior capsule and hip flexors. Pull the uninvolved knee to the chest while supine, simultaneously pushing the involved extremity against the bed.
- Evaluate for assistive devices for the home (shower chair, elevated commode seat, etc.).
- With a straight-back chair, work on sit/stand; increase repetitions as tolerated.
- Continue ambulation 2 times a day with assistance.

1 to 2 weeks

- Discharge criteria:
  1. Gets out of bed independently
  2. Able to ambulate 50 feet in the hall independently with assistive device as necessary
  3. In and out of the bathroom independently
- If discharge criteria are not met or if patient is elderly and lives alone, an extended rehabilitative facility may be appropriate.
- Institute home program with or without outpatient physical therapy (depending on the patient's preinjury activity level). Home exercise program should take the patient only 20 to 30 minutes 2 times per day to ensure compliance.
- Perform quadriceps sets, gluteal sets, ankle pumps, hip and knee active ROM (hip slides in supine), supine abduction of the hip, progressive straight leg raises when tolerated by the patient.

Continued

REHABILITATION PROTOCOL—cont'd

Femoral Neck Fractures, Intertrochanteric Fractures, and Subtrochanteric Fractures

1 to 2
weeks
—cont'd

- Add standing hip abduction, adduction, extension, and flexion, with hip and knee flexion exercises. Include 4-point exercises. This involves flexing the knee while standing, then straightening the knee. Flex the knee again, then return the foot to the starting position.
- Always reinforce good posture while exercising in the standing position.
- Progress ambulation from use of a walker to use of a cane, but the walker should be used as long as the patient has a Trendelenburg lurch, which indicates continued gluteus medius weakness.

- Emphasize gluteal strengthening, especially standing, to improve balance and proprioception. Do exercises on both legs to strengthen both concentric and eccentric components.
- Stationary bicycle, pool exercises, treadmill may be of benefit.

**Special
Considerations**

- Instruct patients with hemiarthroplasty in the use of adduction pillow, hip precautions (adduction, internal rotation, flexion), weight bearing to tolerance (WBTT). (See Chapter 7.)

Femoral Shaft Fractures

A contraindication to intramedullary nailing is contamination so severe that the open fracture wound cannot be converted to a clean contaminated wound, in which case traction or external fixation is used. External fixation may be converted to intramedullary fixation if wound stability is obtained within the first
2 weeks after injury; however, infection is much more likely when intramedullary nailing is performed afterprolonged external fixation or in patients with soft tissue envelopes with infection or drainage.

Technical aspects of intramedullary nailing that affect rehabilitation include the diameter of the nail used, the method of insertion, the mode of interlocking, the amount of fracture comminution, and the severity of soft tissue injuries.

Whether unreamed insertion techniques have any advantages over reamed insertion techniques is still controversial. However, nails inserted without reaming usually are of smaller diameter and have smaller screws than those inserted with reaming. Most authors recommend a decrease in the amount of initial weight bearing when smaller diameter nails are used. Most static-locked 12-mm nails are sufficiently strong to permit unrestricted weight bearing if the fracture is stable with bone-on-bone contact. Partial weight bearing of 50 lbs usually is recommended during phase 1 (0 to 6 weeks) of rehabilitation if smaller diameter nails are used or if fracture comminution or bone loss prevents significant load sharing by the femur.

REHABILITATION PROTOCOL

Femoral Shaft Fracture Treated With Intramedullary Fixation

Phase 1
0 to 6
weeks

- If the fracture has bone-to-bone contact and a *stable* construct with a nail diameter of **12 mm** or more, allow weight bearing to tolerance, with progression to full weight bearing as tolerated, usually by 6 to 12 weeks. For patients with *unstable* fractures or fractures stabilized with **small-diameter nails**, begin with 25 kg ($\approx$ 50 lbs) weight bearing with crutches or walker as other injuries permit.

- Begin quadriceps sets, gluteal sets, hamstring sets, ankle pumps.

- Perform straight leg raising in all planes, supine and standing.

- Perform knee active ROM exercises (flexion and extension).

- Use stationary bicycle for ROM and strengthening.

- Instruct and observe crutch walking technique.

- Begin open- and closed-chain exercises as tolerated.

Phase 2
6 weeks to
3 months

- If full weight bearing is not possible, use a scale technique. The patient places the injured extremity on a scale to measure the amount of weight bearing that is comfortable. Instruct the patient to progress weight bearing in 5- to 10-kg increments each week until full weight bearing is possible. Continue the crutches until the patient can bear full weight in the one-limb stance. Use a cane if necessary until gait is corrected with no lurch or Trendelenburg gait. Most patients regain 80% to 90% of full

Phase 2—cont'd
6 weeks to
3 months
—cont'd

ROM during this phase. With smaller diameter nails (10 to 11 mm), achieve-full weight bearing incrementally using the scale technique for progression.
- Perform isokinetic exercises.
- Perform closed-chain exercises (p. 152).

Phase 3
3 to 6
months

- Most patients have progressed to full weight bearing and from crutches to a cane. If the patient is not full weight bearing and radiographic studies reveal lack of healing, consider either dynamization or bone augmentation (bone grafting, electrical stimulation).
- Continue closed-chain exercises until the patient obtains full knee and hip ROM, can perform a full squat, and can climb and descend stairs full weight bearing without an assistive device.

Thigh circumference should be almost equal to the uninjured side before discontinuing rehabilitation.

Phase 4
>6 months

- Most patients have returned to athletic activities other than contact sports, which must be judged on an individual basis. If a plateau is reached with no improvement in the amount of weight bearing or evidence of nail loosening or screw breakage, and there are signs of radiographic nonunion, exchange nailing or autologous bone grafting may be considered.

CAUTION: If delayed healing is suspected, the patient should be evaluated to rule out occult infection, vascular insufficiency, or metabolic etiology for the nonunion.
- Resume full work and recreational activities as tolerated.

REHABILITATION PROTOCOL

Femoral Shaft Fracture Treated With Plate-and-Screw Fixation

Rehabilitation is the same as that following intramedullary nailing, with the exception that the patient is kept non–weight bearing with crutches for 8 to 12 weeks. Weight bearing is not progressed until evidence of consolidation of the fracture is visible on two radiographic views, usually at 3 to 6 months.

Phase 1
- Begin isometrics and upper extremity conditioning while in traction (preop).

Phase 2
- Apply cast brace or hinged, commercial rehabilitation brace.
- Ambulate with 20 kg weight bearing until evidence of bridging callus on two radiographic views.

- Begin open- and closed-chain exercises (p. 152).
- Perform ROM exercises for knee in cast brace.

Phase 3
- Remove brace.
- Ambulate with crutches until achieving full weight bearing in single leg stance.
- Progress open- and closed-chain exercises (p. 152).
- Stress active ROM and active-assisted ROM of the knee after cast removal.

Distal Femoral Metaphyseal and Epiphyseal Fractures

The most commonly used classification of distal femoral fractures in adults is that of Müller et al. (Fig. 4-4).

These fractures usually require open reduction and internal fixation for restoration of joint congruity.

■ *To avoid loss of reduction and malunion, weight bearing should be delayed for patients with distal femoral intraarticular fractures.*

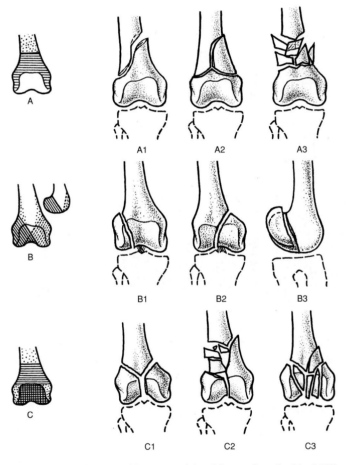

Figure 4-4 Classification of fractures of distal femur described by Müller et al. (Redrawn from Müller ME et al: *The comprehensive classification of fractures of long bones,* Berlin, 1990, Springer-Verlag.) (From Kyle RF: *Fractures of the hip.* In Crenshaw AH, editor: *Campbell's operative orthopaedics,* ed 8, St Louis, 1992, Mosby–Year Book.)

REHABILITATION PROTOCOL

Distal Femoral Intraarticular Fracture With Plate-and-Screw or Intramedullary Fixation

Most patients do not regain full ROM after these injuries and should be advised of this early in the rehabilitation process.

Phase 1
0 to 6 weeks

- Begin active and active-assisted ROM exercises of the knee.
- May use CPM in the first 24 to 48 hours if fixation is sufficiently stable. In general, encourage 0 to 90 degrees of motion.
- Begin open-chain exercises (straight leg raises, quadriceps sets, and short arc quadriceps sets) and continue throughout rehabilitation.
- Allow only touchdown weight bearing.

Phase 2
6 to 12 weeks

- Begin stationary bicycling, minimal to no tension. Allow progression if fixation is stable and radiographs show callus and no fracture gap.
- Begin partial weight-bearing program with crutches or walker at 8 to 12 weeks, using the scale technique (p. 164).
- Begin closed-chain exercises and continue open-chain exercises (p. 152).

Phase 3
3 to 6 months

- Progress to full weight bearing.
- Perform closed- and open-chain exercises (p. 152).

■ *Delayed weight bearing, persistence of pain, and radiographic evidence of fracture gap at 3 to 6 months is an indication for cautious progression of weight bearing and the possibility of a delayed union or nonunion.*

Phase 4
>6 months

- Permit return to work and recreational activities, avoiding excessive squatting, climbing, and jumping. Avoid contact sports for 6 to 12 months, with evaluation of return to contact sports made on an individual basis.

Patellar Fractures

Patellar fractures in adults generally are classified as shown in the box.

Nondisplaced and stable fractures are treated nonoperatively. Functionally, this is indicated by the ability of the patient to extend the knee actively. An inability to extend the knee implies disruption of the extensor mechanism and functional loss, and is an indication for operative treatment. Other indications for operative treatment are comminution that requires total or partial patellectomy and an intraarticular fracture with more than 3 mm of displacement (step-off) of the articular surface. More than 3 mm of displacement or diastasis at the fracture site is a relative indication.

Most current fixation techniques for patellar fractures use a tension band concept that allows early, active knee ROM after the soft tissues are stable. If patellectomy is performed, the retinaculum and extensor mechanism are repaired. Immobilization is continued for 6 to 8 weeks before ROM and closed-chain exercises are begun.

Classification of Patellar Fractures in Adults

Nondisplaced
Transverse
Vertical

Displaced
Transverse
Vertical

Comminuted
Entire patella (patellectomy)
Inferior pole (inferior pole patellectomy)
Superior pole (superior pole patellectomy)

Extraarticular

REHABILITATION PROTOCOL

Patellar Fracture Treated Nonoperatively

0 to 6 weeks	• Wear long-leg cast for 2 to 3 weeks. • Allow weight bearing to tolerance with crutches. • Begin quadriceps sets, gluteal sets, hamstring sets, and straight leg raises in all planes (supine and standing) before discharge from the hospital (quadriceps sets help decrease adhesion formation during the healing process). • May begin open- and closed-chain exercises with the cast on, especially for hip strengthening. • Replace cast with controlled motion brace at 2 to 3 weeks. • Progress weight bearing to tolerance with crutches to weight bearing with the use of a cane. • In general, begin strengthening and ROM exercises at week 3 or 4 (open- and closed-chain exercises).
0 to 6 weeks cont'd	• Begin gentle patellar mobilization; the patient should be independent with this exercise. • Begin scar mobilization to help desensitize the area. • Begin electrical muscle stimulation (EMS) for quadriceps reeducation. • Stationary bicycling with the seat elevated and no resistance is beneficial for ROM and strengthening. Initiate at approximately 6 weeks. • Begin isokinetic exercises at speeds of 60 to 120 degrees per second to strengthen the quadriceps musculature and decrease the forces on the patellofemoral joint that occur at lower speeds. • Use stool scoots for hamstring strengthening. • Continue icing until effusion resolves.

| 6 to 12 weeks | • Begin and progress closed-chain exercises, such as minisquats and step-ups.
• May use a Theraband for resistance in hip exercises and minisquats.
• Start BAPS board exercises.
• Begin lunges.
• Can use stationary bicycling with affected leg only to aid strengthening.
• Since most patients with patellar fractures eventually develop some degree of chondromalacia, emphasize that restoration of quadriceps strength is essential to assist in the absorption of body-weight load that is transmitted up the kinetic chain. | 6 to 12 weeks cont'd | • The exercise program should emphasize restoration of lower extremity strength and flexibility. After this is achieved, implement a maintenance program with emphasis on closed-chain exercises. All exercises should be in a pain-free ROM.
• Evaluate the entire lower extremity, especially for excessive pronation of the feet, which may add stresses to the knee and exacerbate patellofemoral-type symptoms. Use orthotics if excessive pronation is noted. |

Acute Patellar Dislocation

Most acute patellar dislocations are treated with closed reduction and immobilization in a cast or brace. Operative treatment may be necessary if an osteochondral fracture has occurred; any displaced osteochondral fragments are removed, and the disrupted medial tissues, including the vastus medialis muscle, are repaired.

REHABILITATION PROTOCOL

Acute Patellar Dislocation

1 to 7 days	• Decrease edema with ice and elevation. • Begin isometric exercises, quadriceps sets, hamstring sets, gluteal sets, and adductor sets. (Because the vastus medialis obliquus [VMO] fibers originate from the adductor magnus, adductor strength is important in patellofemoral rehabilitation.) • Begin straight leg raises in all directions, with emphasis on adduction. • Evaluation of tight structures and stretching: Iliotibial band may produce a lateral static force on the patella Hamstrings, if tight, may increase the work of the quadriceps during knee extension Gastrocnemius and soleus complex, if tight, may increase pronation during gait, which will increase the dynamic Q angle, causing the patella to track laterally • Perform manual resistive exercises (PNF for strengthening and to assess areas of weakness). • Perform short arc exercises to increase the amount of strength; use of EMS may be helpful. • Use stationary bicycle with the seat high and little to no resistance. • Use VMO biofeedback for VMO strengthening.
2 weeks	• Add weights to straight leg raises. If any pain, decrease the lever arm force by placing the weights around the proximal tibia or the distal thigh. • Increase VMO exercise range from 0 to 20 to 0 to 45 as tolerated and add resistance appropriately.

Continued

REHABILITATION PROTOCOL—cont'd

Acute Patellar Dislocation

2 weeks —cont'd	• Continue stationary bicycle activity, progress to one-legged bicycling. • Use standing hip machine or Theraband for resistance, again with emphasis on hip adduction. • Pool exercises may be beneficial. • Begin closed-chain exercises. • Use BAPS board for ROM and proprioception. • May use accessory weights to emphasize the concentric and the eccentric strength of the VMO.
3 to 6 weeks	• Begin isokinetics at a rate of 120 degrees per second in a pain-free ROM. • May use McConnell taping techniques (see Chapter 5) to assist with normalizing patellar alignment. Placing the patella in better alignment allows the VMO to fire at its optimal length, which increases its strength.

	• Progress closed-chain exercises. • Begin activities with both legs; progress to one-leg exercises, such as minisquats, stand-to-sit exercises, BAPS board, and wall sits. • Begin proprioceptive training with BAPS board and Fitter. • Use stair-climbing machine with short arcs and slow speeds.
6 to 12 weeks	• Continue closed-chain exercises. • Emphasize endurance with agility training as the patient returns to sports. • Consider placing a ¼-in wedge on the medial side under the shoe to decrease foot pronation and decrease stress on the knee while doing minisquats. • Evaluate for excessive pronation secondary to forefoot varus, rearfoot varus, or both. Make appropriate orthosis to correct the abnormalities.

Tibial Plateau Fractures

The Schatzker classification of tibial plateau fractures (Fig. 4-5) has become the most widely used, replacing the earlier Hohl-Moore system.

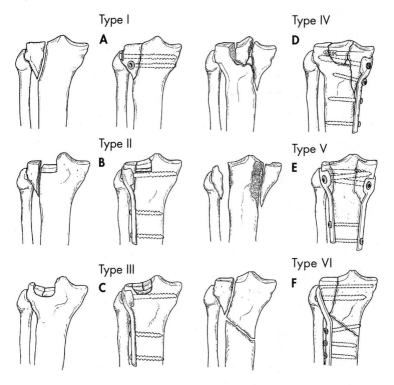

Figure 4-5 A, Type I, pure cleavage fracture. **B,** Type II, cleavage combined with depression. Reduction requires elevation of fragments with bone grafting of resultant hole in metaphysis. Lateral wedge is lagged on lateral cortex protected with buttress plate. **C,** Type III, pure central depression. There is no lateral wedge. Depression may also be anterior, posterior, or involve whole plateau. After elevation of depression and bone grafting, lateral cortex is best protected with buttress plate. **D,** Type IV. Medial condyle is either split off as wedge (type A) as illustrated, or it may be crumbled and depressed (type B), which is characteristic of older patients with osteoporosis (not illustrated). **E,** Type V. Note continuity of metaphysis and diaphysis. In internal fixation both sides must be protected with buttress plates. **F,** Type VI. Essence of this fracture is fracture line that dissociates metaphysis from diaphysis. Fracture pattern of condyles is variable and all types can occur. If both condyles are involved, proximal tibia should be buttressed on both sides. (Redrawn from Schatzker J, McBroom R, Bruce D: *Clin Orthop* 138:94, 1979).

REHABILITATION PROTOCOL

Stable, Local Compression Fracture of the Tibial Plateau

LESS THAN 6-MM DEPRESSION, VARUS/ VALGUS STABILITY	• Begin early ROM (CPM, active assisted). • Keep non–weight bearing for 8 weeks, progressing to full weight bearing by 12 weeks.
GREATER THAN 6-MM DEPRESSION, VARUS/ VALGUS INSTABILITY MORE THAN 10 DEGREES	• Begin early ROM, use CPM. • Use touchdown to non–weight bearing for 8 weeks. Progress slowly to full weight bearing at 12 weeks. • Begin open-chain exercises. • Begin closed-chain exercises when weight bearing is allowed.
STABLE INTERNAL FIXATION POSSIBLE	• Begin CPM in recovery room. • The day after surgery, teach the patient quadriceps sets, hamstring sets, gluteal sets, and straight leg raises in all planes, supine and standing. • Delay weight bearing until healing is evident on radiographs, usually at 8 to 12 weeks. • When weight bearing is allowed, begin closed-chain exercises for the appropriate weight-bearing status of the patient (p. 152).

TIBIAL FRACTURES WITH LIGAMENTOUS INJURY

- May limit ROM initially to allow healing of the ligamentous injury.
- A motion control bracing system is preferable to a typical long-leg cast unless the patient is noncompliant.
- Begin quadriceps sets, hamstring sets, gluteal sets, VMO strengthening, and straight leg raises with a stretching program that includes the hip, knee, and ankle. Tight hip flexors will shorten the involved leg, which is especially a problem if the patient already has decreased extension.

- Begin patellar mobilization techniques (superior, inferior, medial, and lateral).
- Delay full weight bearing for 8 to 12 weeks.
- May begin swimming and stationary bicycling at 8 weeks if clinical evidence of good healing is evident.
- At 8 weeks, continue strength and ROM exercises. Begin a closed-chain exercise program and gradually progress. Begin PWB minisquats and gradually progress to stair-stepping.

REHABILITATION PROTOCOL

Stable Tibial Plateau Fracture or Operatively Stabilized Fracture

Phase 1
0 to 6 weeks

- Use CPM during hospitalization until obtaining 0 to 90 degrees of motion.
- Begin straight leg raises, quadriceps sets, and hamstring sets.
- Begin patellar mobilization techniques (medial, lateral, superior, and inferior).
- Begin active and active-assisted knee ROM exercises (**non**–weight bearing).
- Begin **gentle** passive ROM techniques for extension and flexion, including prone hangs, passive extension with roll under heel, and wall slides while lying supine.

Phase 2
6 to 12 weeks

- Begin progressive weight bearing, depending on fracture-fixation stability and radiographic findings of fracture repair.
- Allow stationary bicycling with minimal or no tension.
- Begin closed-chain exercises, initially with limited weight on affected extremity (8 to 12 weeks) (p. 152).

Phase 3
3 to 6 months

- Progress to full weight bearing and decrease dependence on ambulatory assistive devices in stepwise fashion (crutches–one crutch-cane).

Phase 3 —cont'd 3 to 6 months —cont'd	**Phase 4** >6 months
• Continue open- and closed-chain exercises until thigh and calf circumferences are almost equal to opposite leg. • Unaided stair climbing may be possible. • Return to sedentary or light-duty work.	• Progress work activities as tolerated. May require functional capacity evaluation for moderate to heavy work. • Resume light recreation. No contact sports recommended for 1 year.

Tibial Shaft Fractures

STABLE, LOW-ENERGY TIBIAL SHAFT FRACTURES

Closed reduction is preferred for stable, low-energy tibial shaft fractures. Exceptions include bilateral fractures, floating knee injuries, fractures with intraarticular extension, ipsilateral intraarticular fractures, and fractures in which closed reduction cannot be obtained or maintained. The patient is placed in a long, posterior splint with stirrup strap or a long-leg cast, and radiographs are obtained immediately to evaluate fracture alignment. No distraction of the fracture fragments should be accepted, because distraction of as little as 5 mm has been shown to increase healing time to as much as 8 to 12 months.

HIGH-ENERGY, UNSTABLE, OR OPEN TIBIAL SHAFT FRACTURES

Operative stabilization generally is required for high-energy tibial shaft fractures, many of which are open injuries. Relative indications for operative treatment include failure to obtain acceptable closed reduction, segmental fractures, displaced intraarticular fracture extension into the knee or ankle, bilateral shaft fractures, and fractures with compartment syndrome or vascular injury that requires arterial repair. Fixation may be obtained with plate-and-screw devices, intramedullary nails, or external fixators.

REHABILITATION PRINCIPLES

Postoperative rehabilitation of patients with operatively treated fractures depends on the following factors:

- Open or closed fracture. Open fractures have much higher incidences of delayed union and nonunion and have a poorer prognosis for healing than do closed fractures.
- Extent of injuries associated with open fracture, based on the Gustilo-Anderson classification (p. 149). This classification considers the mechanism of injury (high or low energy); the degree of soft tissue damage; the fracture configuration, comminution, and stability; the level of contamination; and concomitant neurovascular injuries.
- Stability of fracture fixation (strength and type of fixation used)
- Concomitant fractures of the ipsilateral or contralateral lower extremity. Other fractures may change the rate of rehabilitation and the progression of weight bearing.

- Overall medical condition of the patient. Some conditions are associated with delayed fracture healing, such as alcoholism, immunocompromise, and systemic diseases.
- Presence of superficial or deep infection.

OTHER CONSIDERATIONS

- **Bone graft by history.** If bone loss is more than 50% of cortical surface, early bone grafting is recommended at 6 to 8 weeks after the soft tissue environment has stabilized. Autogenous cancellous iliac bone is preferred.
- **Dynamization.** If bony consolidation is not progressing sequentially at approximately 6 weeks, options include removal of the screws from the longest fragment of the fracture to allow dynamization. This allows increased compression at the fracture, contact of the fracture ends, and improved healing. *Removing the screws from the longest fragment increases stability after removal.* If unacceptable shortening is anticipated because of bone loss, the implant should not be dynamized, but should be allowed to remain in static mode and a bone graft should be used.
- **Knee and foot ROM.** Active ROM exercises of the knee and foot should be continued whenever possible throughout the rehabilitation protocol to avoid knee flexion contracture or equinus deformity.
- **Early stabilization** of fractures in patients with multiple injuries reduces the incidence of pulmonary complications (adult respiratory distress syndrome, fat embolism, and pneumonia), decreases the number of days in the intensive care unit, and shortens the hospital stay (Bone et al.).
- The **rate of rehabilitation** may be slowed in type III wounds by soft tissue considerations. Anderson found that type III fractures averaged 3 months until soft tissue healing was complete. Soft tissue stability is aided by use of constructs such as foot mount on external fixators.

REHABILITATION PROTOCOL

Stable, Low-Energy Tibial Shaft Fracture Treated With Closed Reduction and Casting

0 to 3 weeks	• Begin quadriceps sets, hamstring sets, gluteal sets, and straight leg raises in all planes before discharge from the hospital. • Strongly encourage early weight bearing to tolerance on crutches. Use of a shoe lift for the contralateral extremity will aid in swing-through with a long, straight leg cast. • Make radiographs 7 to 10 days after reduction to check fracture alignment.
3 to 5 weeks	• Swelling should be diminished enough to allow careful fitting of a PTB cast or short leg cast. • Increase weight bearing as tolerated.
	• Begin active AROM exercises of the knee, 0 to 140 degrees. Perform straight leg raises and quadriceps sets several times a day, in addition to other open-chain exercises. • May use Theraband or ankle weights to add resistance. • Begin closed-chain exercises according to weight-bearing status.
6 to 8 weeks	• Patient should be ambulating weight bearing as tolerated in the PTB or short leg cast. • Continue open- and closed-chain exercises for the hip and knee. • Continue hip and knee ROM.

2 to 4 months

- Discontinue PTB or short leg cast when clinical evidence of complete healing is present (average healing time is 4 months). Determine healing with radiographic appearance and lack of tenderness on palpation and ambulation.
- Begin ankle stretching, ROM, and strengthening exercises.

- Continue progressive strengthening exercises, including leg presses, Stair-master, lunges, toe raises, bicycling, and treadmill, until calf and thigh circumferences are equal to uninjured extremity.

■ *If fracture reduction is lost and alignment becomes unacceptable during weight bearing, the fracture probably should have been stabilized initially with an intramedullary nail. Treat loss of reduction with reduction and fixation with an intramedullary nail or biplanar external fixator.*

REHABILITATION PROTOCOL

Open Tibial Shaft Fracture Treated With Unreamed, Static Interlocked Intramedullary Nail

Phase 1
0 to 6 weeks

- Apply PTB or short leg cast.
- Patients with 8-mm or 9-mm nail begin touchdown weight bearing with crutches or walker.
- 10-mm nails or larger allow partial weight bearing with crutches.
- Begin active and passive knee ROM exercises.
- Begin quadriceps sets, VMO sets, short arc quadriceps exercises (open chain).
- Begin closed-chain exercises according to weight-bearing status (p. 152).

Phase 2
6 weeks to 3 months

STABLE FRACTURE
- Discontinue cast if early callus is present.
- Start ankle and subtalar ROM, continue knee therapy (active ROM plus towel stretches).
- Progress to weight bearing as tolerated with crutches.
- Progress closed-chain rehabilitation.

TYPE III OPEN FRACTURE
- Consider *"bone graft by history"* at 6 weeks, or eventual exchange nailing at 8 to 12 weeks, for 8- or 9-mm nail if no callus is visible or continued bone defect is present.

Phase 3
3 to 6 months

- Progress to weight bearing as tolerated with crutches.
- Dynamize (remove distal or proximal screws) if minimal evidence of healing and gap present at fracture.
  NOTE: remove screws that are the greatest distance from fracture.
- Consider bone graft if no fracture gap and evidence of delayed healing in open fracture.
- If the fracture is united, progress to cane, then to independent ambulation.
- Resume functional activities and begin agility training; return to sports as tolerated.

Phase 4
>6 months

- If ununited, treat for **delayed union/ nonunion** with exchange nailing, bone graft, electrical stimulation, or fibular osteotomy.
- Rule out biologic problem, such as infection or vascular insufficiency.

REHABILITATION PROTOCOL

Tibial Shaft Fractures Treated With Biplanar Hexfix External Fixation

Stable Open Fractures

Phase 1
0 to 6 weeks

- Begin partial weight bearing with crutches (30 lbs).
- Begin knee and hip ROM exercises (open chain).
- Cover soft tissue at 5 to 7 days.
- Begin closed-chain rehabilitation according to weight-bearing status.

Phase 2
6 weeks to 3 months

- If soft tissues are stable, apply PTB cast or long-leg cast after fixator removal.
- If soft tissues are unstable, maintain and dynamize (see p. 181) external fixator; remove foot mount attachment when soft tissues are stable.

Phase 3
3 to 6 months

- Continue with open-chain exercises and progress with closed-chain exercise.
- If minimal callus, consider bone grafting.

Phase 4
6 months

- If healing is not progressing, treat as delayed union (see nonunion guidelines, p. 181).
- Do *not* use intramedullary nail fixation because of high incidence of infection with intramedullary nailing after external fixation.

Unstable Tibial Fractures (Closed and Open Types I and II)

Phase 1
0 to 6 weeks

- Begin touchdown weight bearing with crutches.
- Perform hip and knee ROM exercises (open chain).
- Stabilize foot with foot-mount attachment to control soft tissue motion in open fractures (especially distal third fractures).

Phase 2
6 weeks to 3 months

- Remove foot mount and dynamize frame (p. 181).
- Begin aggressive active and passive ROM of ankle and knee: SLRs, quadriceps sets, VMO exercises, short arc quadriceps sets.
- Progress weight bearing with crutches.
- Continue open-chain exercises and begin closed-chain rehabilitation.

Phase 3
3 to 6 months

- Begin weight bearing to tolerance with crutches.
- Perform bone graft if evidence of delayed healing.
- Ensure frame is properly dynamized.
- Progress closed-chain rehabilitation.

Phase 4
>6 months

- If no evidence of healing, treat for delayed union (p. 181).

Unstable Tibial Fracture (Open Type III)

Phase 1
0 to 6 weeks

- Begin touchdown weight bearing with crutches.
- Stabilize foot with foot-mount attachment on all frames for soft tissue stability.
- Begin hip and knee ROM exercises.

■ Note: Be aware of the type of coverage used. For example, a free flap may not "take" if too much movement in the area decreases wound stability.

Continued

REHABILITATION PROTOCOL—cont'd

Tibial Shaft Fractures Treated With Biplanar Hexfix External Fixation

Unstable Tibial Fractures (Closed and Open Types I and II)—cont'd

Phase 2
6 weeks to 3 months)

- Bone graft by history at 6 weeks:
  Posterolateral—preferred because of good blood supply and better incorporation of bone graft; skin usually better.
  Posteromedial—often indicated in proximal fourth of tibia (where peroneal nerve makes posterolateral approach difficult).
  Anteromedial—skin must be in good condition.
- Slowly progress weight bearing over several weeks.
- If gap present at fracture, manually compress fracture in office or at time of surgery.

- Remove foot mount.
- Perform aggressive ankle and knee ROM exercises.
- Continue open-chain and begin closed-chain exercises.

Phase 3
3 to 6 months

- Begin weight bearing to tolerance with crutches.
- Dynamize fixator (see p. 181).
- Progress closed-chain rehabilitation.

Phase 4
>6 months

- If no evidence of healing, treat as delayed union or nonunion (p. 181).

Tibial Shaft Fracture Treated With Biplanar Ilizarov External Fixation

Phase 1

0 to 6 weeks

- Begin partial weight bearing as tolerated.
- In general, keep patients with intraarticular fractures at partial weight bearing at 30 to 50 lbs for 4 to 6 weeks (Fig. 4-6).
- Allow patients with nonarticular injuries to be weight bearing to tolerance.

■ *Patient must be at least partially weight bearing before discharge from hospital to avoid contracture.*

- Begin aggressive exercises for ankle and knee ROM: ankle pumps, ankle inversion and eversion exercises, SLRs, quadriceps sets, VMO exercises (open chain, p. 152).

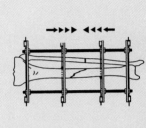

Figure 4-6 Ilizarov-type fixation of tibia and fibula.

Continued

Tibial Shaft Fracture Treated With Biplanar Ilizarov External Fixation

Phase 1 —cont'd
0 to 6 weeks —cont'd

- Retighten frame bolts before discharge from hospital.
- Use walking shoe and Theraband for dorsiflexion stretching to prevent equinus contracture if foot mount is not used.
- Use towel stretches for passive dorsiflexion of ankle.
- Begin closed-chain rehabilitation according to weight-bearing status.

Phase 2
6 weeks to 3 months

- Begin weight bearing to tolerance.
- Maintain wire tension and treat pin-tract infection aggressively.

Phase 3
3 to 6 months

- Evaluate for contractures and treat as necessary with passive ROM and active ROM exercises.
- Advance closed-chain rehabilitation.
- If evidence of delayed healing, compress fracture ¼ turn for 20 days.

Phase 4
>6 months
DELAYED UNION

- Ensure frame stability, revise and replace wires as necessary.
- Watch closely for pin-tract problems.
- Biologic treatment: bone graft or compression/distraction.
- Apply splint to avoid equinus contracture, if needed.

PREVENTION OF CONTRACTURES WITH THE USE OF ILIZAROV-TYPE EXTERNAL FIXATION

Contractures may be avoided by stretching exercises, night positioning, splinting, and functional use of the extremity.

Passive stretching exercises for the calf and hamstring muscles should be done 2 to 3 hours each day. Calf stretching should include towel stretches, runners' stretch, use of an incline board, and use of rubberbands for dorsiflexion.

■ *Passive exercises are far more effective in preventing contractures than are active exercises.*

Night positioning is helpful in preventing contractures by changing the patient's usual sleeping posture. Most patients with an Ilizarov-type fixator choose a position that places the foot in plantar flexion and the knee in flexion. Patients are taught to place a pillow under the most distal ring of the fixator to keep the knee extended and to wear a shoe with the foot tied in dorsiflexion to the frame.

Both static and dynamic splinting have a role in the management of patients with Ilizarov-type fixation. *Static splints* include fixed-position orthoses (AFO foot mount), straps, ropes, and other nonelastic devices to hold the foot out of equinus (in neutral). These devices are especially helpful at night, when the constant pressure of a dynamic splint may be too uncomfortable to allow sleep. *Dynamic splints* may be as simple as an elastic band from the shoe to the fixator. More elaborate devices include a spring-loaded, clamp-on dynamic extension splint.

Functional use of the extremity is important not only to prevent contractures, but also to encourage bone regeneration. Weight bearing is strongly encouraged. An obstacle course provides good motivation for younger patients. Retro walking on a treadmill decreases the amount of dorsiflexion needed in the gait. The amount of dorsiflexion needed can be controlled by increasing the incline of the treadmill. As ROM improves, the incline height can be gradually decreased until the patient is able to walk forward. This allows patients without full dorsiflexion to increase weight bearing on the involved leg and to ambulate without pain or limp.

CHAPTER FIVE

The Knee

S. BRENT BROTZMAN, MD
PENNY HEAD, PT

Anterior Cruciate Ligament Reconstruction

REHABILITATION RATIONALE

Rehabilitation after reconstruction of the anterior cruciate ligament (ACL) has changed significantly in recent years, with protocols becoming increasingly aggressive. Despite changes in protocol design, however, the goal of rehabilitation has remained the same: to return the patient to a preinjury level of activity. This involves restoration of normal range of motion (ROM), strength, and stability of the knee to allow return to functional activities. In athletes, the rehabilitation program must also strive to restore agility, skill, and speed, as well as a functionally stable knee that can withstand all rigors of sports-related activities.

After ACL reconstruction, the proper balance between protection of the reconstructed ligament and prevention of disuse sequelae may be difficult. The reconstructed ligament must be properly protected to allow healing and to prevent excessive strain on the graft; however, prolonged immobilization is not desirable because of the numerous detrimental effects associated with this form of treatment, including disuse atrophy of muscle tissue, severe changes in articular cartilage and ligaments, and the loss of joint ROM from the formation of intraarticular adhesions.

Although numerous rehabilitation protocols have been based on clinical observations of ACL patients, a relative paucity of research exists to provide basic scientific information on how rehabilitation affects the reconstructed ligament *in vivo*. "Accelerated" rehabilitation programs have recently become widely used, despite their apparent divergence from accepted biomechanical and histologic principles. These accelerated protocols are based on the observation that patients who did not comply with the restrictions imposed by a traditional protocol had better ROM, strength, and function without compromising joint stability than did those who complied.

Rehabilitation programs continue to progress as new information becomes available about factors affecting the reconstructed ligament. Although no definitive ACL protocol has been universally agreed on as the most effective, most current protocols stress the following principles:

- Initiation of early ROM and weight bearing
- Early edema control techniques
- Avoidance of excessive stress to the graft (avoiding excessive *early* open-chain exercises)
- Early hamstring strengthening to provide dynamic joint stability and to decrease strain on the graft
- Proprioceptive retraining and neuromuscular reeducation.

- Muscle strengthening and conditioning
- Incorporation of closed kinetic chain exercises
- Sports-specific agility training
- Aerobic cardiovascular training
- A bracing algorithm
- Criteria-based progression from one level to the next
- Criteria-based return to athletic activity

BASIC SCIENCE AND BIOMECHANICS

■ *In early stages of healing, failure of the ACL graft usually occurs at the site of fixation, rather than in the graft itself.*

For an in-depth discussion of the basic science and biomechanics of ACL reconstruction, please refer to *Clinical Orthopaedic Rehabilitation.*

REHABILITATION CONSIDERATIONS

Preoperative Rehabilitation

Preoperative rehabilitation of acute ACL injury should focus on the following:

- Decreasing joint effusion
- Restoring full ROM
- Strengthening the quadriceps and hamstrings
- Restoring a normal gait pattern

Joint effusion usually can be controlled with limb elevation, cryotherapy, compression, and modalities such as high-voltage galvanic stimulation (HVGS); however, aspiration also may be required. It is extremely important to diminish joint effusion because of its neuromuscular inhibitory effects on the quadriceps, which result in rapid atrophy of the quadriceps muscles.

Several studies report an increased incidence of *arthrofibrosis* after reconstruction of an **acutely** injured ACL. Shelbourne et al. noted a decreased incidence of arthrofibrosis by delaying surgery at least 3 weeks. We delay ACL reconstruction until the patient has regained full ROM with minimal to no pain. This avoids the risk of loss of motion associated with attempting to rehabilitate a swollen knee with an acutely inflamed, painful synovium.

Early Motion in an "Accelerated" Protocol

Historically, patients with ACL reconstructions were treated with prolonged immobilization to protect the graft tissue. This conservative form of treatment resulted in numerous complications, such as intraarticular adhesions, joint stiffness, patellofemoral crepitus and pain, and profound quadriceps weakness. Eriksson and Haggmark demonstrated 40% quadriceps atrophy after just 5 weeks of immobilization. In addition, the rate of atrophy was increased with immobilization in a shortened position (such as joint flexion).

■ *The hallmark of accelerated rehabilitation protocols is an emphasis on aggressive, early accomplishment and long-term maintenance of full knee extension.*

The goals for ROM in an accelerated protocol, according to Fu et al., are full knee extension (equal to the uninvolved knee) within 2 to 3 weeks after surgery and full flexion within 8 weeks.

Reducing Stress on the ACL Graft

The current trend of accelerated ACL rehabilitation appears to diverge somewhat from the established basis of science and rehabilitation principles. To minimize postoperative complications, such as arthrofibrosis and quadriceps atrophy, ACL rehabilitation has become more aggressive; however, this aggressive rehabilitation must be performed in a manner that minimizes inflammation and avoids excessive loading on the reconstructed ligament.

Closed Kinetic Chain (CKC) Exercises Versus Open Kinetic Chain (OKC) Exercises

Knee exercises for rehabilitation after ACL reconstruction are divided into two broad categories: open kinetic chain and closed kinetic chain.

Closed kinetic chain (CKC) exercises are those in which motion at the knee is accompanied by motion at the hip and ankle. The distal segment of the extremity (foot) is in contact with a pedal, platform, or ground surface. Examples of CKC exercises include minisquats (Fig. 5-1), cycling, and leg presses.

CKC exercises promote cocontraction and increase stability through increased joint compressive loads. Cocontraction minimizes the anterior translation of the tibia on the femur that occurs with increased compressive loads, thus reducing shear forces on the joint and strain on the ACL. Because of reduced strain on the ACL, CKC exercises can be incorporated early in the rehabilitation program to strengthen the quadriceps.

Open kinetic chain (OKC) exercises are those in which motion at the knee is independent of motion at the hip and ankle. The distal segment of the extremity (foot) is free to move. Examples of OKC exercise include leg extensions and leg curls.

OKC quadriceps exercise, e.g., Kin-Com quadriceps strengthening, often is avoided early in ACL rehabilitation because of the significant stress it places on the reconstructed ligament. Numer-

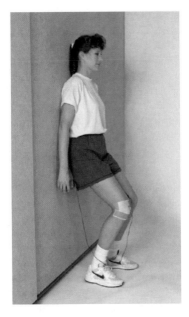

Figure 5-1 Minisquats performed against wall initially (wall sits). Patient does not flex beyond 30 degrees. These are later performed without a wall.

ous studies have demonstrated that OKC quadriceps exercises through a full ROM may damage the graft. This form of exercise isolates quadriceps activity, thus increasing anterior translation of the tibia and placing excessive strain on the ACL graft from 30 degrees flexion to full extension.

OKC quadriceps exercise can be used in a restricted ROM, avoiding the last 30 to 45 degrees of knee extension, to allow the isolated quadriceps strengthening that is necessary to restore normal strength and muscle girth.

OKC hamstring curls can be performed early in the rehabilitation program because they decrease the level of strain on the ACL throughout the entire ROM. Because the hamstrings are the primary dynamic stabilizers of the knee, early initiation of hamstring strengthening should be emphasized.

Active, isolated quadriceps contraction in a non–weight-bearing position (OKC), places undesirable shearing stress on the reconstructed ligament by increasing anterior translation of the tibia on the femur. When external resistance as low as 7 lbs. is applied to the distal tibia, the quadriceps force required to extend the leg is almost 2 times the force required with no resistance. This significantly increases the stress on the reconstructed ACL.

■ *Shearing stress on the ACL is greatest from 30 degrees of flexion to full extension.*

This stress can be neutralized either by simultaneous, isometric contraction of the hamstrings with the quadriceps (cocontraction), in either an open- or closed-chain fashion, or by avoiding open-chain quadriceps exercises between 0 to 45 degrees of flexion. This restriction of ROM avoids isolated quadriceps contraction in the zone of greatest ACL stress.

Cocontraction of the hamstrings with the quadriceps (such as in minisquats or leg presses) adds a posterior translatory force to counteract anterior translation induced by the quadriceps; therefore, cocontraction is thought to stabilize the knee during the strengthening process. Many ACL protocols avoid active-resisted isolated quadriceps strengthening for several months after ACL reconstruction because of the potential stress on the graft. Instead, they incorporate CKC exercises to promote cocontraction of the hamstrings and quadriceps to protect the graft during strength training. The hamstrings are the primary dynamic stabilizers of the knee, acting synergistically with the ACL, as well as protecting it from excessive stress. Reestablishing a hamstring/quadriceps strength ratio that is equivalent to or higher than that of the unoperated limb has produced better functional outcomes after ACL reconstruction.

Another advantage of CKC exercises is the significant decrease in patellofemoral joint forces compared with those generated by OKC quadriceps exercises in the range of 60 to 90 degrees of knee flexion. CKC quadriceps exercises generally are performed with the knee in nearly full extension, thus avoiding one of the most common pitfalls of ACL rehabilitation: the patellofemoral pain syndrome. Paulos' "paradox of exercise" is successfully avoided by using CKC quadriceps strengthening instead of OKC exercises from 60 to 90 degrees.

Arthrofibrosis

Several studies report a frequent occurrence of arthrofibrosis after reconstruction of an acutely injured ACL. Shelbourne et al. suggest that delaying surgery at least 3 weeks from the time of injury significantly decreases the incidence of arthrofibrosis. ACL reconstruction should be delayed until the patient has regained full ROM of the knee with only minimal pain. Postoperative rehabilitation of a knee with an acutely inflamed, painful synovium may increase the risk of LOM.

Electromyogram (EMG) Biofeedback

EMG biofeedback transforms myoelectric signals produced by the muscle into visual and/or auditory signals for the patient. A threshold or goal is set by the therapist for the patient to try to obtain. Once the patient produces a strong enough muscle contraction to exceed the threshold level, the visual and/or auditory signals occur. The threshold can then be raised to elicit a stronger contraction by the patient.

A common use for EMG biofeedback is to improve contraction of the vastus medialis obliqus (VMO) (Fig. 5-2). When joint effusion inhibits quadriceps activity, research indicates that the VMO "wastes first and wastes most." Because it is the only medial dynamic stabilizer of the patella, weakness of the VMO results in patellar maltracking, which may lead to patellofemoral pain syndrome.

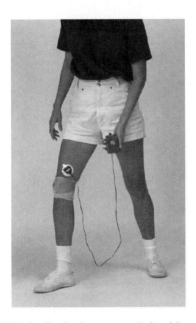

Figure 5-2 EMG biofeedback of vastus medialis oblique (VMO) muscle to improve quality of contraction.

ACL BRACING

Knee braces are classified into four categories: prophylactic, rehabilitative, functional and transitional. Please see *Clinical Orthopaedic Rehabilitation* for bracing recommendations.

CRITERIA FOR RETURN TO SPORTS

Return to sports activity is the usual goal after ACL reconstruction. Several different guidelines have been established to help determine when an athlete may safely return to sports; these guidelines vary among rehabilitation protocols.

Paulos and Stern

Paulos and Stern recommend a return to sports when the following criteria are met:
- Minimum of 9 months after surgery
- No swelling
- Completed jog/run program
- Isokinetic testing of the quadriceps indicates 85% strength compared with uninvolved leg
- Isokinetic testing of the hamstrings indicates 90% strength compared with uninvolved leg
- Single leg hop for distance test 85% of uninvolved leg
- Full ROM (0 to 140 degrees)

Although recognizing that the efficacy of bracing for graft protection is questionable, Paulos and Stern use a functional ACL brace during sporting activities for 1 year after surgery. They use a 20-degree extension stop in the brace to limit the limb to 7 to 10 degrees of extension.

Andrews and Wilk

Andrews and Wilk recommend a return to sports at 5 to 6 months after surgery if the following criteria are met:
- Isokinetic testing of quadriceps and hamstrings fulfills criteria
- KT-1000 test unchanged from initial test
- Functional test 80% or greater compared with contralateral leg
- Proprioceptive test 100% of contralateral leg
- Satisfactory clinical exam

The criteria for isokinetic test results, as well as what types of functional and proprioceptive tests are used, are not given by the authors.

Shelbourne and Nitz

Shelbourne and Nitz recommend a return to sports at 4 to 6 months after surgery if the following criteria are met:

- Isokinetic test indicates quadriceps strength is greater than 80% of the contralateral leg at 60, 180, and 240 degrees per second
- Full ROM
- No joint effusion
- Satisfactory ligament stability test using the KT-1000
- Successful completion of functional progression

Shelbourne and Nitz recommend the use of a functional ACL brace up to 1 year after reconstruction.

Frndak and Berasi

Frndak and Berasi recommend a return to sports when the following criteria are met:
- Minimum of 9 months after surgery
- Full ROM
- Isokinetic test indicates quad strength at least 90% of uninvolved leg
- No pain or swelling
- Successful completion of preathletic agility training

Campbell Clinic

At the Campbell Clinic, therapists use the following guidelines to determine when an athlete can return to sport:
- Full ROM
- No joint effusion
- Isokinetic test indicates quadriceps strength is 80% or more than uninvolved leg
- Isokinetic test indicates hamstring strength is 85% or more than uninvolved leg
- One-legged hop for distance test is 85% compared with uninvolved leg
- Successful completion of running program
- Successful completion of sports-specific agility program
- Satisfactory clinical exam

Return to sport varies between 6 and 12 months, depending on the surgeon's preference. The use of an ACL functional brace also depends on the surgeon's preference.

Rehabilitation After Central Third Patellar Tendon ACL Reconstruction

The following section provides descriptions of several established ACL protocols. Both traditional and accelerated protocols are presented.

The semitendinosus tendon protocol (Table 5-3) is progressed slower in consideration of the weaker initial fixation, greater graft compliance, and slower soft tissue–to–bone healing after the use of these grafts.

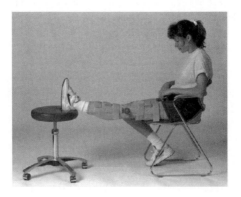

Figure 5-3 Extension of knee on stool.

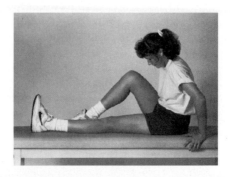

Figure 5-4 Quadriceps sets.

REHABILITATION PROTOCOL

ACL Reconstruction CAMPBELL CLINIC

The Campbell Clinic protocol (Table 5-1) emphasizes early ROM, weight bearing, and functional rehabilitation similar to the Shelbourne protocol; however, it is not considered to be as aggressive in terms of the timing of certain activities and return to sporting activity.

0 to 2 weeks	• During the initial postoperative period, emphasize decreasing joint effusion, improving quadriceps control, and obtaining full knee extension (Fig. 5-3).
	• Initiate quadriceps setting (QS) in full knee extension (Fig. 5-4) on the first postoperative day to prevent neurophysiologic shutdown of the quadriceps muscles; continue until 3 to 4 weeks.
	• Initiate straight leg raises in all planes when the patient can perform a QS sufficient to prevent an extensor lag (Fig. 5-5).

Add ankle weights when the patient can correctly perform 3 sets of 10 to 15 repetitions with ease. Progress the weights according to patient's tolerance. Begin active hamstring curls, prone and standing, early in the rehabilitation progression.
- Perform passive ROM exercises, such as towel extensions (Fig. 5-6), on postoperative day 1 to obtain full knee extension.
- As pain subsides, use prone leg hangs to promote or maintain full extension (Fig. 5-7). Perform passive ROM for knee flexion to 90 degrees by sitting on the edge of the bed and lowering the involved extremity with the uninvolved extremity (Fig. 5-8).

Continued

REHABILITATION PROTOCOL—cont'd

ACL Reconstruction CAMPBELL CLINIC

TABLE 5-1 Campbell Clinic ACL Rehabilitation Protocol—ACL Reconstruction

| | Weeks | | | | | Months | | | |
	1-2	3-4	5-6	7-8	9-12	4	5	6	7-12
Bracing									
Straight leg immobilizer/motion control brace (MCB) at 0 degrees	X	X							
Functional brace with exercise/sport			X	X	X	X	X	X	X
Range of Motion									
Braced in extension except with exercise	X	X							
Prone hangs/towel extension	X	X	X	X	X				
Knee flexion out of brace	X								
90 degrees		X							
120 degrees			X						
Full flexion (135 to 140 degrees)			X						
Weight Bearing									
50% weight bearing	X								
75% to 100% weight bearing		X							
Discontinue crutches		X							
Delay weight bearing with meniscal repair			X						

Strengthening								
Quad sets/SLR (all planes)	X	X						
Stool scoots	X	X						
Wall sits	X	X	X	X	X	X	X	
Hamstring curls (prone/standing)		X	X	X	X	X	X	X
Multihip machine			X	X	X	X	X	X
Progressive closed-chain activities			X	X	X	X	X	X
Knee extension (90 to 60 degrees)/proximal resistance	X		X	X	X	X		
Knee extension (90 to 40 degrees)/proximal resistance			X	X	X	X	X	
Knee extension (full range)				X	X	X	X	X
Conditioning								
Stationary bike—low resistance	X	X						
Stationary bike—progress resistance			X	X	X	X	X	X
Outdoor bike				X	X	X	X	X
Treadmill (forward/retro)			X	X	X	X	X	X
Stairmaster/cross-country ski machine				X	X	X	X	X
Jogging/running					X	X	X	X
Agility/Sport-Specific Training								
Fitter/slide board				X	X	X	X	X
Resisted running with SportCord					X	X	X	X
Plyometric training						X	X	X
Carioca, cutting, figure 8's, etc.						X	X	X

REHABILITATION PROTOCOL—cont'd

ACL Reconstruction   CAMPBELL CLINIC

0 to 2 weeks —cont'd	• When the patient is able to achieve 80 to 90 degrees of flexion, initiate wall slides (Fig. 5-9). • Begin patellar mobilizations Figs. 5-10 and 5-11, especially superior gliding, during this initial postoperative period. • Use electrical stimulation for neuromuscular reeducation if the patient demonstrates a poor QS on initial evaluation by the physical therapist. • Bracing and weight bearing depend on the surgeon's preference and the surgical procedure performed. Typically, the patient is placed in a straight leg immobilizer or a rehabilitative brace, allowing 0 to 90 degrees of motion. The brace or immobilizer may be removed to perform ROM exercises several times throughout the day. The brace can also be removed for showering or bathing once the incisions have healed. • Allow weight bearing to tolerance with crutches if the brace is locked in full extension; the patient remains non–weight bearing if concomitant meniscal repair is performed. Encourage a normal, symmetric gait.
2 to 4 weeks	• Open the brace to allow full ROM. • Continue to emphasize maintenance of extension using prone leg hangs, towel extensions, and passive ROM by the therapist if indicated. • Knee flexion should progress to 120 degrees by the end of 4 weeks. • Add weights to prone and standing hamstring curls as tolerated.

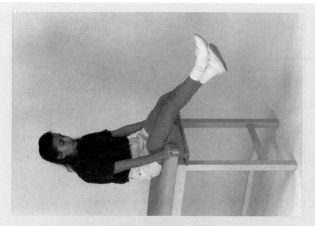

Figure 5-8 Passive flexion of the knee.

Continued

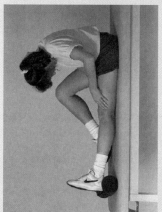

Figure 5-6 Patient places heel on rolled towel to aid in knee extension. Patient may be instructed to push downward on quadriceps with the hands to passively increase extension.

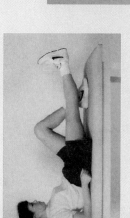

Figure 5-5 Straight leg raise.

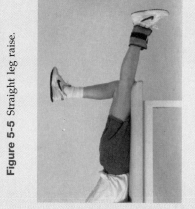

Figure 5-7 Prone leg hangs to increase knee extension.

REHABILITATION PROTOCOL—cont'd

ACL Reconstruction   CAMPBELL CLINIC

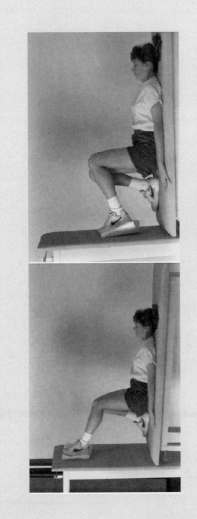

Figure 5-9 Wall slides aid with knee flexion by utilizing gravity to assist flexion. The patient slowly slides the foot down the wall until a sustained stretch is felt in the knee.

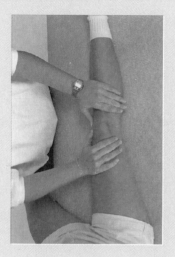

Figure 5-11 The patella is mobilized medially, laterally, and especially superiorly.

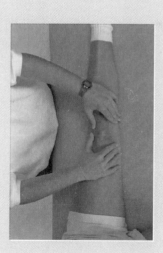

Figure 5-10 Patellar mobilization to avoid contractures (e.g., patella infera).

Continued

REHABILITATION PROTOCOL—cont'd

ACL Reconstruction CAMPBELL CLINIC

2 to 4 weeks —cont'd

- Also progress weights with the SLR program. Once the patient can lift 10 lbs in each direction, use the multihip machine for hip strengthening.
- Initiate the stationary bicycle during week 2 if knee flexion ROM is adequate. Use minimal resistance early in the bicycling program.
- Initiate closed kinetic chain (CKC) exercises at 2 weeks after surgery, unless concomitant meniscal repair is performed. These exercises include minisquats and leg presses, beginning with both legs and progressing to a single leg as tolerated (Fig. 5-12).
- Initiate wall sits, another form of CKC exercise, at a 45-degree angle (see Fig. 5-1). It is important to make sure the patient's tibia remains vertical during this exercise to prevent excessive stress to the graft. The patient progresses the exercise by increasing the sitting time.
- Begin proprioceptive training early with the BAPS board, starting with two legs and progressing to one; and progress weight-shifting activities to one-legged stance (Fig. 5-13).
- Begin lateral step-ups on a 2- to 4-inch step when the patient can perform single leg minisquats. Progress this exercise by increasing the height of the step as strength improves (Fig. 5-14).
- Begin ambulation on the treadmill (forward and retro) between 2 and 3 weeks with emphasis on a normal gait. A mirror may be used to provide visual feedback during ambulation.

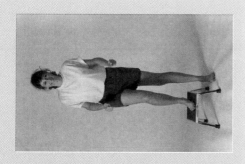

Figure 5-12 Leg press.

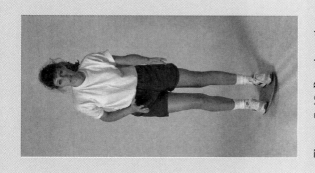

Figure 5-13 Proprioception with BAPS board.

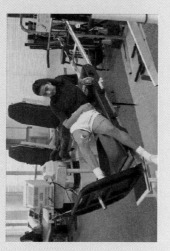

Figure 5-14 Lateral step-ups. Patient stands on a stable stair step. The operated leg is bent slowly, lowering the opposite foot to the floor. Return to the starting position.

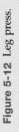

Continued

REHABILITATION PROTOCOL—cont'd

ACL Reconstruction CAMPBELL CLINIC

2 to 4 weeks —cont'd	• Perform submaximal active knee extension in the 90- to 60-degree range, with manual resistance by the therapist. • Progress to full weight bearing without crutches when patient can ambulate without a limp. This usually occurs by the third or fourth postoperative week.
	to 40 degrees, with the tibial pad placed proximally. At 6 weeks, employ higher speed isokinetic quadriceps work in conjunction with the isotonic training; the range is still limited to 90 to 40 degrees, and the pad is still proximal. • The typical procedure is to fit the patient for an ACL functional brace at 6 weeks postoperatively, depending on the surgeon's preference.
4 to 6 weeks	• Full ROM should be achieved by 6 weeks. • Continue to emphasize full knee extension. • May begin use of stairmaster or Nordic-Track cross-country ski machine. • Continue to progress strengthening program according to patient's tolerance. • Begin hamstring progression from isotonics to isokinetics on the Kin-Com. • Also use the Kin-Com for quadriceps strengthening in the isotonic mode from 90	
8 to 10 weeks	• Progress all of the above exercises, and add lunges (Fig. 5-15). • Initiate slow-form running with the Sport-Cord (forward and retro). • Continue isokinetic quadriceps work at various speeds. • Begin lateral strengthening and agility at 10 weeks using the Fitter and the slide board (Fig. 5-16).

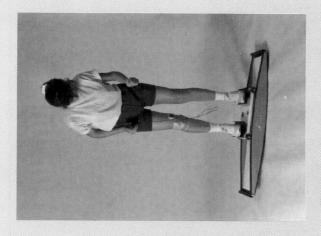

Figure 5-16 Fitter for lateral agility.

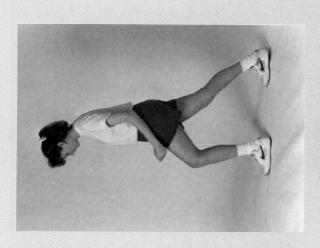

Figure 5-15 Lunges.

Continued

REHABILITATION PROTOCOL—cont'd

ACL Reconstruction CAMPBELL CLINIC

12 weeks	• Allow full-range isotonics for the quadriceps on the Kin-Com; move the tibial pad to midrange. Progress isokinetic quadriceps work to full extension by 16 weeks postoperatively. • Begin the knee extension machine with emphasis on low weight and high repetitions. • Initiate slow, controlled lateral SportCord drills. • Continue progression of the strength program. • Perform an isokinetic evaluation of hamstring strength. If the test indicates hamstring strength is 85% or better, discontinue isokinetic hamstring workouts; however, encourage the patient to continue hamstring workouts on the machines.
16 to 18 weeks	• Evaluate quadriceps strength isokinetically; retest the hamstrings if necessary. • Institute a jogging program and a plyometric program if quadriceps strength is at least 65% of the uninvolved extremity, no effusion is present, the patient has full ROM, and the knee is stable.
5 to 6 months	• Begin agility training and sports-specific drills if the above criteria have been met. • Perform retesting of the quadriceps if necessary. • Return to sport depends on the surgeon's preference; however, the patient must exhibit at least 80% quadriceps strength and 85% hamstring strength (see p. 201). • If a functional brace was prescribed by the surgeon, it is usually recommended that it be worn for sporting activity for at least 1 year after surgery.

ACCELERATED REHABILITATION PROTOCOL

ACL Reconstruction SHELBOURNE AND NITZ

This four-phase rehabilitative protocol emphasizes early restoration of full knee extension (equal to the uninvolved knee), immediate weight bearing, and closed-chain exercises (Table 5-2). Although the protocol is accelerated in terms of early full extension, quadriceps activity, and early return to athletic play, the term accelerated does *not* apply to the initial 2 weeks after surgery.

During the first 14 days of postoperative rehabilitation, the patient focuses on five goals: full extension, wound healing, good quadriceps leg control, minimal swelling, and flexion to 90 degrees. Allow weight bearing to tolerance with the assistance of crutches, but encourage the patient to be up and about only for bathroom privileges and meals. During the remainder of this time, encourage the patient to limit walking and to elevate the limb. Shelbourne and Nitz believe that this initial 2 weeks of rest greatly decreases postoperative swelling, therefore allowing faster advancement toward normal activities of daily living and earlier return to sports activity.

Phase 1 This phase actually begins shortly after the acute knee injury and weeks before the reconstructive surgery. The initial focus is on regaining ROM and decreasing joint effusion. A CryoCuff (Aircast, Summit, NJ) is used to provide both cooling and compression in the attempt to decrease swelling. Patients also work on restoring a normal gait pattern during this phase. Once swelling and pain are decreased and full ROM is restored, begin strengthening exercises.

Phase 2 The second phase of the accelerated protocol encompasses the initial 2 weeks after surgery. Place the patient in a straight leg immobilizer immediately after surgery; also apply the CryoCuff. Begin the use of CPM once the patient returns to the hospital room on postoperative day 1 and continue until discharge *Continued*

REHABILITATION PROTOCOL—cont'd

ACL Reconstruction SHELBOURNE AND NITZ

TABLE 5-2 Shelbourne and Nitz Accelerated ACL Rehabilitation Protocol

	Weeks					Months			
	1-2	3-4	5-6	7-8	9-12	4	5	6	7-12
Bracing									
Straight leg immobilizer/MCB at 0 degrees	X								
Functional brace with exercise/sport		X	X	X	X	X	X	X	X
Range of Motion									
Braced in extension except with exercise	X								
Passive range of motion (PROM) for full knee extension	X	X	X						
CPM	X	X							
Knee flexion ROM	X	X	X						

Weight Bearing							
Weight bearing to tolerance with crutches	X						
Full weight bearing without crutches		X					
Strengthening							
Quadriceps sets/SLR (all planes)	X	X	X	X	X	X	X
Active knee extension (90 to 30 degrees)	X	X	X	X	X	X	X
Calf raises		X	X	X	X	X	X
Minisquats/step-ups		X	X	X	X	X	X
Progressive closed-chain activities			X	X	X	X	X
Conditioning							
Biking	X	X	X	X	X	X	X
Swimming	X	X	X	X	X	X	X
Stairmaster		X	X	X	X	X	X
Running (if strength test 70%)				X	X	X	X
Agility/Sport-Specific Training							
Lateral shuffles			X	X	X	X	X
Cariocas			X	X	X	X	X
Jumping rope					X	X	X

REHABILITATION PROTOCOL—cont'd

ACL Reconstruction SHELBOURNE AND NITZ

Phase 2 —cont'd

from the hospital, on the second or third postoperative day. Use the CPM for 10 minutes every hour with the heel of the operative extremity propped on pillows to allow full knee extension. Place a 2.5-lb ankle weight on the proximal tibia to help promote full knee extension. Also begin PROM for terminal knee extension and for knee flexion to 90 degrees out of the CPM.

The patient begins working on leg control on the first postoperative day. This is done by using active quadriceps setting and straight leg raising. Perform the above exercises for knee flexion/extension PROM and leg control 3 times a day during the initial 2 weeks. Also perform active quadriceps contractions in the range of 90 to 30 degrees.

Allow weight bearing to tolerance with crutches immediately after surgery; however, encourage patients to

limit activity to meals and bathroom privileges during the first 2 weeks.

After discharge from the hospital, usually on postoperative day 2, patients continue with PROM, leg control exercises, and active knee extension 90 to 30 degrees. Initiate prone leg hangs and towel extensions (see Fig. 5-7) at week 1 to maintain or promote full knee extension. Begin wall slides (see Fig. 5-9), heel slides (Fig. 5-17), and active-assisted flexion to promote knee flexion ROM.

During the second week after surgery, it is permissible for patients to return to classes or light office work on a part-time basis, depending on the amount of swelling in the knee.

Use the straight leg immobilizer during the initial 2 weeks after surgery when the patient is out of the house. It is not required when ambulating around the house. At follow-up evaluation by the surgeon at 7 days postoperatively, measure the patient for a functional brace without blocks to extension or flexion. This brace replaces the immobilizer after the initial 2 weeks and works as a protective device during inclement weather and when the patient is returning to athletic activity.

Phase 3 This phase of rehabilitation usually encompasses 3 to 5 weeks postoperatively. Emphasize a normal gait pattern without the use of crutches, as well as a gradual return to normal activities of daily living. Full knee extension with minimal swelling continues to be a primary focus. Encourage the restoration of normal knee flexion; patients typically achieve full flexion (135 degrees) 5 weeks postoperatively.

May initiate strengthening exercises, such as calf raises, minisquats, leg presses, and step-ups (see p. 217), between 2 and 3 weeks postoperatively. Patients may also begin using the Stairmaster, bicycling, and swimming.

Continued

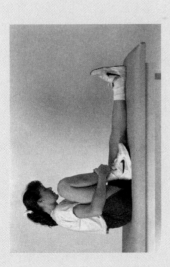

Figure 5-17 Heel slides.

TABLE 5-3
Semitendinosus Protocol (Lonnie Paulos, MD)

Activities/Daily Living	Week								Month					
	1	2	3	4	5	6	7	8	3	4	5	6	9	12
Shower without brace				◄──────────────────────────►										
Sleep without brace						◄──────────────────►								
Break down brace						◄──────────────────►								

Extension
- Lie on stomach and lower leg into extension
- Sit on firm surface and place 5 to 10 lbs above knee

Flexion
- Lie on back; use gravity to slide foot down wall
- While sitting use gravity and opposite leg to bend knee

Range of Motion	Week							
	1	2	3	4	5	6	7	8
Passive								
Extension/flexion	10/70	10/70	10/70	9/90	9/100	9/110	9/120	Full
Active								
Extension/flexion	30/60	30/60	25/70	20/80	15/90	10/100	5/110	0/120

Brace Settings	Week								Month					
	1	2	3	4	5	6	7	8	3	4	5	6	9	12
Weight bearing						50%	75%	100%	Full ◄──────────────────────────►					

Knee-brace ROM setting
- Brace locked at 30 degrees for first 2 weeks postoperatively
- Unlock brace to exercise angles after 2 weeks postoperatively

				Week								Month		
	1	2	3	4	5	6	7	8	3	4	5	6	9	12
For exercise														
Extension/flexion	30/60	30/60	25/70	20/80	15/90	10/100	5/110	0/120	Open					
For ambulation														
Extension/flexion						20/100	20/110	20/120	D/C'd for walking at twelfth week					
Strength Training														
Quad sets, SLRs (brace locked at 40 degrees)	← week 1 → week 8													
Electrical stimulation (brace locked at 40 degrees)	← week 1 → week 8													
Hamcurls			← week 3 → month 12											
Total hip	← week 1 → week 8													
Minisquat/leg press/toe rise						← week 6 → month 12								
Cycling—stationary					← week 5 → month 12									
Cycling—outdoor			Level ground only							Seated hill climb		Standing hill climbs		

Continued

TABLE 5-3—cont'd
Semitendinosus Protocol (Lonnie Paulos, MD)

Balance/Coordination	Week								Month					
	1	2	3	4	5	6	7	8	3	4	5	6	9	12
Baps/KAT/Sandunes/Rhomberg/tape touch								→→→→→→→→→→→→→→→→→→						↑
Profitter									→→→→→→→→→					↑
SportCord lateral agility									→→→→→→→→→					↑

Conditioning	Week								Month					
	1	2	3	4	5	6	7	8	3	4	5	6	9	12
Cycle with well leg		→→→→→→			↑									
UBE (upper body ergonometer)	→→→→→→→→→→→→→→→→→→→→→→→													↑
Swimming (refer to pool protocol)					20° →→→→→→→→→→→→→→→									↑

	Week								Month					
	1	2	3	4	5	6	7	8	3	4	5	6	9	12
Walking (100% weight)								10°	→	→	→	→	→	→
Stairmaster									20°	→	→	→	→	→
Cross-country ski machine									20°	→	→	→	→	→
Rowing									30°/90°	→	→	→	→	→
Run/jog (sports brace must be worn)												20°	→	→
Power Training														
Low repetitions—leg press/squats/hamcurls								20°/90°	→	→	→	→	→	→
Isokinetics (refer to protocol)														

To Return to Sports:
- Minimum of 9 months postoperatively
- No swelling
- Complete jog/run program
- Quadriceps strength 85% of opposite knee
- Hamstring strength 90% of opposite knee
- Hop distance 85% of opposite knee
- ROM 0 to 140 degrees

Modified from Jackson DW: *The anterior cruciate ligament: current and future concepts,* New York, 1993, Raven Press.

REHABILITATION PROTOCOL—cont'd

ACL Reconstruction SHELBOURNE AND NITZ

Phase 4 The final phase of the accelerated protocol begins at 5 weeks after surgery. Perform an isokinetic strength evaluation with a 20-degree extension block at 180 and 240 degrees per second. If strength testing shows that the involved extremity has reached at least 70% of the strength of the uninvolved extremity, institute a running program. The patient may also begin lateral shuffles, cariocas, and jumping rope. It is also permissible to implement sports-specific agility training. Continue strength training, as well as bicycling, swimming, and/or using the Stairmaster.

Throughout this phase, temper aggressive activity by the control of swelling and the maintenance of ROM. It is noted by Shelbourne et al. that if the patient does not desire a rapid return to sport, a near-normal level of strength will be restored through normal activities of daily living over 1 to 2 years. If the patient does desire a rapid return to sport, intensify strength training in this final phase.

At 10 weeks, perform another isokinetic evaluation at 60, 180, and 240 degrees per second. Perform a KT-1000 to assess ligament stability. Increase agility workouts.

At 16 to 24 weeks, repeat the isokinetic evaluation; allow return to sports if strength is greater than 80% and functional progression has been successfully completed.

Patients can perform most of the rehabilitation on their own. Patients are followed at 1, 2, 5, 9, and 15 weeks postoperatively by both the physician and the physical therapist. During these visits, the therapist guides the patient in progression of exercises and activity. Perform additional follow-up at 6 and 12 months.

COMPLICATIONS/TROUBLESHOOTING

Loss of Motion

Loss of motion, or arthrofibrosis, is recognized as one of the most common postoperative complications following ACL reconstruction. As stated earlier, loss of motion is defined by Fu et al. as a knee flexion contracture of more than 10 degrees and/or knee flexion ROM less than 125 degrees.

It is important to begin passive full knee extension exercises early in the rehabilitation program to prevent scar tissue formation in the intercondylar notch. These exercises, such as prone leg hangs and towel extensions, should be performed until maintenance of full knee extension is assured.

Patellar mobilization, especially superior gliding, should be initiated immediately to prevent shortening of the patellar tendon and decreased patellar mobility.

Mobilization of the tibiofemoral joint may also be necessary to promote knee flexion and extension ROM. Early edema control is important to prevent induration of the peripatellar soft tissues. Induration of these tissues may lead to decreased patellar mobility with resulting loss of motion. Joint effusion may also be exacerbated by an aggressive strengthening program. Nonsteroidal antiinflammatory medication (NSAIDs), as well as modification of the rehabilitation program, may be necessary until the effusion can be controlled.

Infrapatellar contracture syndrome may develop if a fibrous hyperplasia of the anterior soft tissues of the knee occurs. The fibrous hyperplasia entraps the patella and limits knee motion. Early detection of this condition is necessary to prevent significant complications. Signs and symptoms include induration of the peripatellar tissues, painful ROM, restricted patellar mobility, extensor lag, and a "shelf sign."

Patients with unacceptable motion, defined by Graf and Uhr as a flexion contracture of 10 degrees or more or a limitation of flexion of less than 130 degrees, are treated initially with aggressive physical therapy. The use of a Dynasplint (Dynasplint Systems) may be considered; this device produces a low-load prolonged force on restricted soft tissues to restore ROM. If conservative measures fail, patients are treated surgically. At less than 6 months postoperatively, Graf and Uhr and Paulos et al. recommend closed manipulation of the knee, with arthroscopic lysis of adhesions and debridement of the intercondylar notch as necessary. At more than 6 months after surgery, open debridement is recommended.

Patellofemoral Pain

Patellofemoral pain may be caused by flexion contracture, prolonged immobilization, quadriceps weakness, or aggressive open-chain (OKC) quadriceps exercises.

Shelbourne and Nitz found fewer problems with patellofemoral pain symptoms in patients undergoing accelerated ACL rehabilitation, probably because of the initiation of early ROM and CKC quadriceps exercise.

OKC quadriceps strengthening should be performed in a pain-free ROM to prevent exacerbation of patellofemoral pain. Generally, OKC quadriceps exercises in the 90- to 60-degree range produce the highest forces on the patellofemoral joint. A low-weight/high-repetition program should be emphasized with quadriceps exercise if the patient complains of patellofemoral pain.

The use of CKC strengthening decreases the amount of force at the patellofemoral joint. CKC exercises are generally performed near full extension, thus avoiding the increased compressive forces generated from 90 to 60 degrees.

Patellar Tendonitis

Wilk et al. reported that patellar tendonitis is not caused by harvest of the patellar tendon graft. They suggest that if meticulous procurement of the graft is performed, followed by immediate motion and weight bearing, patellar mobilization, and quadriceps strengthening, complications such as patellar tendonitis can be avoided.

Patients often develop symptoms of patellar tendonitis with the initiation of aggressive quadriceps strengthening. It is important to monitor patients for such symptoms, so that a chronic inflammatory process does not ensue. If treated in the acute phase with NSAIDs, ice-cup massage, flexibility exercises, and a reduction or modification of the quadriceps strengthening program, patellar tendonitis generally can be reversed. Some clinicians advocate eccentric quadriceps strengthening in the treatment of patellar tendonitis. Once in the chronic phase, patellar tendonitis becomes harder to treat and can hinder the patient's progress with rehabilitation.

ACL RECONSTRUCTION WITH CONCOMITANT MENISCAL REPAIR

Rehabilitation protocols for the ACL reconstructed knee with concomitant meniscal repair vary according to surgeons' preferences and surgical consideration.

Medial and Lateral Collateral Ligament Injury of the Knee

REHABILITATION RATIONALE

Medial collateral ligament (MCL) injuries usually are caused by a valgus stress. The most common mechanism is a blow to the lateral aspect of the knee. The examiner must make sure, by examination or magnetic resonance imaging (MRI), that concomitant injuries of the knee are not present. The classic O'Donoghue triad of injury is MCL, ACL, and peripheral medial meniscus, but more recent reports indicate that the most common triad is MCL, ACL, and lateral meniscal tear. Isolated MCL injury should be treated nonoperatively, but concomitant intraarticular ligament injuries (ACL) typically require surgical reconstruction. Meniscal pathology also requires surgical intervention. Seventy percent to 80% of patients with acute ACL disruptions present with significant traumatic effusion. The incidence of significant knee effusion with isolated MCL tears is significantly lower (usually 1+ rather than 4+).

Examination

To test for MCL injury, a valgus stress is applied with the knee in full extension and then with the knee in 30 degrees of flexion (Fig. 5-18). As the knee moves into extension, the role of secondary restraints other than the MCL increases. Isolated MCL tear is indicated by instability only at 30 degrees of flexion. Instability in full extension indicates that secondary restraints are disrupted in ad-

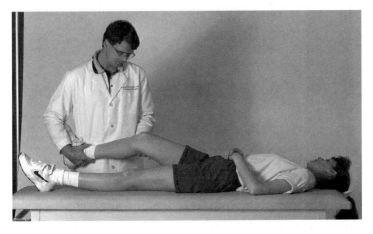

Figure 5-18 Testing of MCL injury with the knee in 30 degrees of flexion. Valgus stress is placed across the knee.

TABLE 5-4 **Severity of MCL and LCL Tears**

Grade	Opening on Exam	MCL/LCL Test	Instability
1	0 to 5 mm	Minimal	None
2	5 to 10 mm	Partial	Some
3	10 to 15 mm	Significant	Moderate
4	Greater than 15 mm	Complete	Grossly unstable

Modified from Miller M: *Review of orthopaedics,* Philadelphia, 1992, WB Saunders.

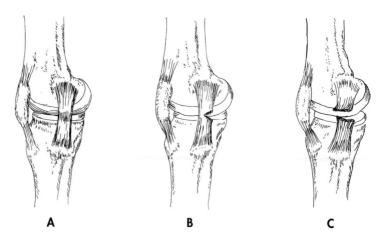

A   **B**   **C**

Figure 5-19 Medial collateral tears of the knee. **A,** Grade 1; **B,** Grade 2; **C,** Grade 3.

dition to the MCL. Tenderness to palpation usually is present over the tibial or femoral attachment. The severity of MCL and lateral collateral ligament (LCL) tears is based on a standard system (Table 5-4 and Fig. 5-19).

Treatment

Isolated MCL tests are treated nonoperatively with protective bracing, early ROM, and physical therapy. Grades 1 and 2 injuries are treated with immediate ROM. Grade 3 injuries are kept non–weight bearing and the brace is locked for 2 to 3 weeks. Chronic instability may require reconstruction using the semi-membranosus tendon (Slocum procedure) or advancing the tibial MCL (Mauck procedure).

For grade 3 MCL tears, many authors advocate locking the brace at 45 degrees of flexion for 2 to 3 weeks, followed by bracing in restricted ROM (0 to 90 degrees). The patient remains non–weight bearing with crutches for 3 weeks. During this immobilization period, isometric exercises (SLRs, quadsets, etc.) are performed. Gentle active ROM exercises may be performed in the brace as tolerated, but restricted weight bearing is continued for 3 months.

LCL injuries usually are caused by a varus stress. Rehabilitation after LCL injury is similar to that after injury of the MCL, but slower healing of LCL usually requires a longer period of brace protection. Complete LCL tears often are managed by operative repair, with or without augmentation with the biceps tendon.

■ *It is important for optimal long-term results that the patient obtain adequate ROM and muscle strength before returning to full activities, including competitive sports. Because individuals heal at different rates, these prerequisites are critical.*

REHABILITATION PROTOCOL

Grades 1 and 2 Injuries of the Medial Collateral Ligament
BROTZMAN AND ROSS

Phase 1

- Apply sturdy rehabilitation brace with settings locked from 15 to 90 degrees.
- Begin partial weight-bearing ambulation with crutches.
- Exercise in brace 3 times daily:
  Isometrics (SLRs, quadriceps sets, VMO exercises)
  Ankle ROM exercises
  Active knee flexion to 90 degrees
  Hip flexion
  90 to 45 degree knee extension
  Hip extension
  Well leg and upper body exercises (aerobic conditioning)
- Remove brace only to shower.
- Use icing (cryotherapy) compression dressings early.
- Prescribe oral NSAIDs.

Phase 2
3 weeks

- Perform exercises out of brace.
- Progress knee flexion and extension, TKE, 90 to 0, side step-ups.
- Begin progressive resistive exercises (PREs) 1 to 10 lbs.
- Begin bicycling when ROM is sufficient.
- Progress partial weight bearing to full weight bearing, no crutches.

Phase 3
6 weeks

- Initiate negative-resistive work.
- Perform PREs with heavy weight.
- Use stationary bicycle.
- Allow functional activities, including straight-ahead running.
- Advance to stadium steps and figure-eight running.

Return to sports

- Confirm painless, stable ROM with no pain on palpation of ligament.
- Ensure absence of effusion or instability.
- Ensure presence of symmetric muscle strength with uninvolved extremity.

REHABILITATION PROTOCOL

Lateral Retinacular Release SHERMAN

1 day	• Begin ROM exercises and knee strengthening the day of surgery.
	• Allow weight bearing as tolerated with crutches, typically using crutches 1 to 2 weeks.
	• Use cryotherapy, compressive wraps, and galvanic stimulation for at least 72 hours for edema control.
	• Employ capsular mobilization techniques by manipulation of patella to prevent recurrent scarring of the surgical release or suprapatellar adhesions (Fig. 5-34).
	• Begin quadriceps strengthening:
	  Straight leg raises
	  Quadriceps sets
	
	Initiate submaximal exercises at terminal extension, progressing to maximum contraction of the VMO as soon as the patient is able.
	• Initiate PREs as tolerated.

2 days	• Begin active-assisted and passive ROM exercises for restoration of full flexion. Begin in the sitting position, then use prone techniques to place the lateral capsular attachments on greater stretch. • Focus on VMO strengthening over next weeks, using VMO biofeedback if required. • Progress PREs. • Continue formal outpatient physical therapy for a minimum of 3 months with active encouragement. *Continued*

REHABILITATION PROTOCOL—cont'd

Lateral Retinacular Release   SHERMAN

Progression of activity:

1. Unassisted walking
2. Swimming
3. Distance walking and cycling
4. Jogging
5. Running
6. Pivoting activities

Program parameters:

- With program adherence, 90% of patients can perform an isometric straight leg raise without an extensor lag and have at least 90 degrees of flexion with minimal effusion at 1 week.
- All patients should have greater than 120 degrees of flexion at 4 weeks.

Iliotibial Band Friction Syndrome of the Knee in Runners

REHABILITATION RATIONALE

Iliotibial band friction syndrome is the most common cause of lateral knee pain in runners. The iliotibial band is a thickened strip of fascia that extends from the iliac crest to the lateral tibial tubercle, receiving part of the insertion of the tensor fasciae latae and gluteus maximus. A bursa and subsequent inflammatory response develop between the band and bony prominence with repetitive flexion and extension of the knee (such as in downhill running). Usually an inflammatory reaction develops between the iliotibial band and the lateral femoral epicondyle (Fig. 5-20); less often the band is irritated at the lateral tibial prominence.

Factors that contribute to the development of iliotibial friction band syndrome include the following:

- Cavus feet   Increases lateral stresses at iliotibial band

- Varus knee position   Increases lateral stresses at iliotibial band

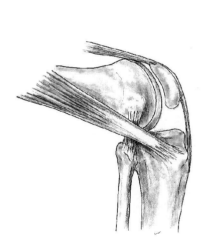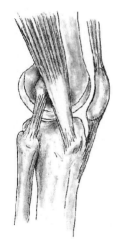

Figure 5-20 As the knee moves from flexion to extension, the iliotibial tract passes from behind to move in front of the lateral femoral epicondyle. The pain experienced by runners with iliotibial tract friction syndrome is caused by the tight band rubbing over the bony prominence of the lateral epicondyle. (Redrawn from Dugas R, D'Ambrosia R: Causes and treatment of common overuse injuries in runners, *J Musculoskel Med* 3(8):113, 1991.)

- Downhill running

  Especially aggravates symptoms because the knee is maintained in a flexed position for longer periods than on a flat surface

- "Downhill" leg on a pitched running surface

  Runners who run consistently on roads that have a drainage pitch often develop iliotibial band friction syndrome of the downside leg (Noble and Clancy)

- Hard shoes, hard surfaces

  Hard running shoes are defined as those having a rearfoot and forefoot impact rating of more than 10 gm and 13 gm, respectively, as tested in 1981 *Runner's World* shoe survey. Hard surfaces include paved roads, but not dirt roads.

Clinical features of iliotibial band friction syndrome include pain and palpable tenderness over the lateral femoral condyle about 2 cm above the joint line during exercise. Pain is exacer-

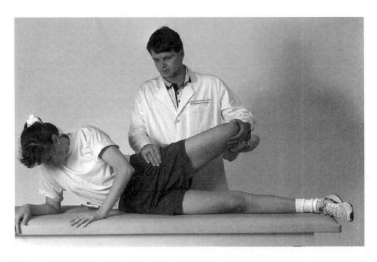

Figure 5-21 Ober's test to detect tightness in the iliotibial tract and tensor fasciae latae muscle. Patients are instructed to lie on their sides. The examiner places the upper leg in abduction and some extension so that the iliotibial band crosses the greater trochanter. The knee may be flexed or extended, the latter stretching the iliotibial band more. The pelvis is stabilized and the upper leg is adducted (lowered) toward the floor. With a tight iliotibial band, the leg remains abducted. If normal, the leg adducts (lowers) to the table surface.

bated by downhill running and often is aggravated by repetitive flexion-extension movements (walking down stairs, running, cycling, or skiing). Usually pain becomes so severe that it limits the athlete to a particular distance. Many patients have iliotibial band tightness, which is diagnosed with Ober's test (Fig. 5-21).

Natural History
Clancy reports that most runners with iliotibial band friction syndrome must rest from running for 6 weeks. Our experience indicates that severe inflammation often requires 6 to 8 weeks of rest before symptoms subside and the patient is able to return to running. Patients with acute or mild symptoms usually respond quickly to conservative measures. For recalcitrant symptoms, Noble recommends surgical release of the posterior fibers of the iliotibial band where they overlie the femoral condyle.

REHABILITATION PROTOCOL

Iliotibial Band Friction Syndrome in Runners

- Rest from running until asymptomatic.
- Ice area before and after exercise.
- Prescribe oral NSAIDs.
- Ensure relative rest from running and high flexion-extension activities of the knee (cycling, running, stair descent, skiing).
- Avoid downhill running.
- Avoid running on pitched surfaces with a pitched drainage grade to the road.
- Use soft running shoes rather than hard shoes (see p. 234).
- Use iontophoresis if helpful.
- Give a steroid injection into the bursa if required.

- Perform stretching exercises:
  Iliotibial band stretching
    Two-man Ober stretch (Fig. 5-22)
    Self–Ober stretch (Fig. 5-23)
    Lateral fascial stretch (Fig. 5-24)
    Posterior fascial stretch plus gluteus maximus and piriformis self stretch (Fig. 5-25)
    Standing wall lean for lateral fascial stretch (Fig. 5-26)
  Rectus femoris self stretch (Fig. 5-27)
  Iliopsoas with rectus femoris self-stretch (Fig. 5-28)
- Use lateral heel wedge in the shoe, especially for those with iliotibial band tightness (Clancy and Noble).
- Build in correction in the shoe for a short leg (leg-length discrepancy) if present.

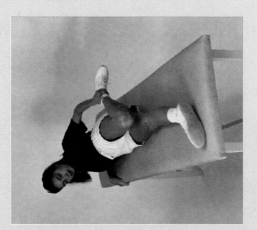

Figure 5-22 Two-man Ober stretch.

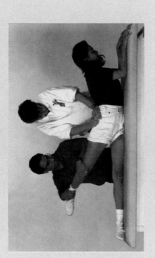

Figure 5-23 Self-Ober stretch.

Continued

REHABILITATION PROTOCOL—cont'd

Iliotibial Band Friction Syndrome in Runners

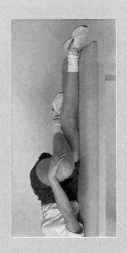

Figure 5-25 Posterior fascial stretch, plus gluteus maximus and piriformis stretch.

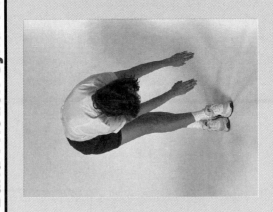

Figure 5-24 Standing lateral fascial stretch. The involved leg is crossed behind the uninvolved leg.

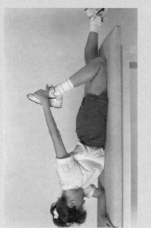

Figure 5-27 Rectus femoris self-stretch.

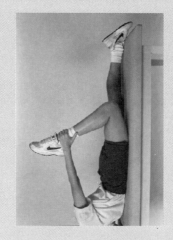

Figure 5-28 Iliopsoas with rectus femoris stretch. Thigh is off the table.

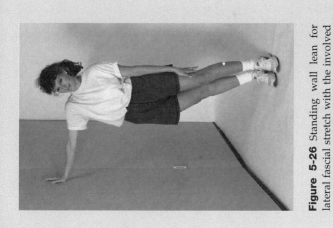

Figure 5-26 Standing wall lean for lateral fascial stretch with the involved leg closest to the wall.

Patellofemoral Disorders

REHABILITATION RATIONALE

Patellofemoral dysfunction, or disorder, may be defined as pain, imbalance, inflammation, and/or instability of any component of the extensor mechanism of the knee. These conditions may result from congenital, traumatic, or mechanical stresses (Shelton and Thigpen).

A careful clinical history and physical examination should be performed to accurately identify the exact syndrome causing the anterior knee pain.

An individual with patellofemoral pain experiences increased pain when the knee is flexed because the patellofemoral joint reaction force (PFJRF) increases with flexion of the knee from 0.5 times body weight during level walking to 3 to 4 times body weight during stair climbing and 7 to 8 times body weight during squatting (Fig. 5-29),

CHONDROMALACIA PATELLAE

There is some confusion in the literature caused by the (incorrect) interchangeable usage of the terms chondromalacia patellae and anterior knee pain. Chondromalacia patellae is a pathologic de-

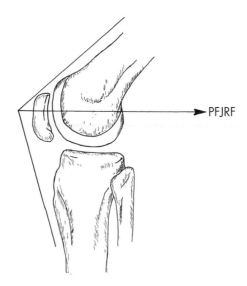

Figure 5-29 Increased patellofemoral joint reaction force (PFJRF) with knee flexion during squatting.

scription of softening of the articular cartilage on the undersurface of the patella. This does not include the other structures involved in anterior knee pain: the patellar tendon, medial and lateral retinacular structures, and intraarticular structures.

Chondromalacia generally is described in the following four stages:

Stage 1   Articular cartilage shows only softening or blistering.

Stage 2   Fissures appear in the cartilage.

Stage 3   Fibrillation of cartilage occurs, causing a "crab-meat" appearance.

Stage 4   Full cartilage defects are present; subchondral bone is exposed.

PATELLAR TILT VERSUS PATELLAR SUBLUXATION

Patellar tilt and subluxation also are entities separate from patellofemoral pain. Chronic patellar tilt tends to be associated with retinacular tightness and pain because the retinaculum is placed under significant tension with knee flexion.

If a line extending from the lateral articular facet of the patella is parallel to or converges with a line from the lateral condyle of the patellofemoral groove, an abnormal condition exists indicative of increased lateral pressure (Fig. 5-30) (Kramer). In contrast, many patients with a lax extensor retinaculum experience frequent patella subluxation without retinacular pain, but they are more prone to instability problems and dislocation.

PATELLAR FUNCTION AND MECHANICS

The patella links the divergent quadriceps muscle to the common tendon, increasing the quadriceps lever arm and thus its mechanical advantage (McConnell, Ficat). To function efficiently the patella must be properly aligned so that it remains in the trochlear groove of the femur. The ability of the patella to track properly in

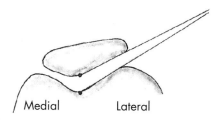

Medial   Lateral

Figure 5-30 Patellar tilt causing an increased pressure on the lateral portion of the patellofemoral surface.

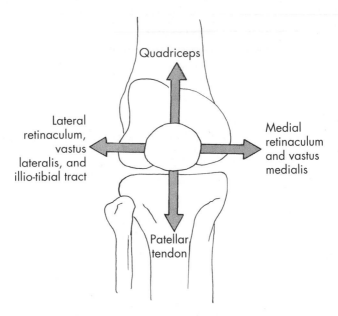

Figure 5-31 Forces around the patella.

Factors Affecting Patellar Alignment (McConnell)

- Increased Q angle
- VMO insufficiency
- Tight lateral structures
- Patella alta: the "superiorly" riding patella rides above the stabilizing structures of the trochlear groove

the trochlear groove depends on the bony structures and the balance of forces of the soft tissues about the joint. Patellar malalignment caused by altered mechanics predisposes an individual to patellofemoral pain.

Lateral forces at the patellofemoral joint are restricted by the medial retinaculum and the VMO; during knee flexion, these are aided by the prominent orientation of the lateral trochlear facet (Fig. 5-31). Any imbalance in these forces may result in patellar maltracking (see box above).

Q angle

The Q angle is formed by the intersection of the line of pull of
the quadriceps and the patellar tendon measured through the center of the patella. A line is drawn from the anterosuperior iliac
spine through the center of the patella and a second line is drawn
from the tibial tubercle to the center of the patella (Fig. 5-32). The
Q angle is normally less than 10 degrees in men and 15 degrees
in women. The upper limit for a normal Q angle is 13 to 15 degrees. An increased Q angle may be associated with increased
femoral anteversion, external tibial torsion, and lateral displacement of the tibial tubercle that increases the lateral pull of the patella.

TREATMENT

The literature reports good results in 75% to 85% of cases with
nonoperative treatment of patellofemoral disorders (Whitten-
becker et al.). Specified periods for conservative trials range from

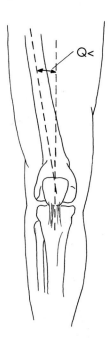

Figure 5-32 Q angle. The Q angle measurement is used to assess the angular alignment of the extensor mechanism. The upper limit of normal is
15 degrees. This angle is formed by the bisection of a line drawn along
the femoral shaft and another drawn along the patellar tendon, from the
tibial tubercle to the center of the patella.

2 to 6 months. We believe a 6-month trial of conservative treatment is warranted to avoid surgical intervention if at all possible.

REHABILITATION CONSIDERATIONS

The most successful rehabilitation programs customize the specifics of the program to the patient. The regimen should allow progression without increasing symptoms. Low exercise intensity and high repetitions help achieve this end. Strength, flexibility, endurance, proprioception, and functional training are the key components of the therapeutic exercise program. Medication, relative rest, external support (taping or Palumbo brace), and modalities are helpful adjuncts.

Strengthening

Strengthening programs are directed at increasing the strength of the VMO muscle. This muscle exerts a stabilizing medial force on the patella, predominantly in the last 30 degrees of extension. (Radin, Fulkerson, and Hungerford). The VMO realigns the patella medially and is the only dynamic medial stabilizer.

Isometric exercises such as QS and straight leg raises are most frequently used for strengthening. These exercises produce smaller

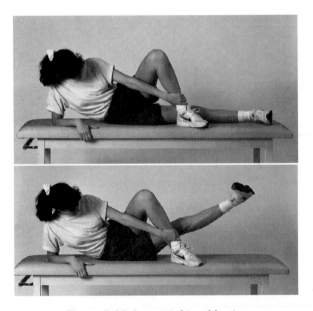

Figure 5-33 Isometric hip adduction.

PFJRF than larger arc exercises and usually are less painful. Soder-berg and Cook demonstrated that the rectus femoris was most ac-tive during straight leg raises and that the vastus medialis, biceps femoris, and gluteus medius were most active during QS. VMO biofeedback is a useful adjunct in helping the patient properly iso-late the VMO (see Fig. 5-2).

The use of hip adductor contractions in conjunction with QS and straight leg raises have been recommended to facilitate VMO strengthening because of the VMO origin near the adductor mag-nus (Shelton and Thigpen) (Fig. 5-33). Terminal knee extension ex-ercises (SAQ exercises) also are used to improve quadriceps strengthening in the least efficient portion of the arc of motion (Shelton and Thigpen). Closed-chain strengthening techniques are encouraged. Eccentric ankle dorsiflexion exercises have been re-ported to reduce patellar tendonitis symptoms. (Shelton and Thig-pen)

Results of EMG recordings of the VMO are shown in Table 5-5.

Flexibility

Flexibility training has been strongly emphasized as a component in the treatment of patellofemoral disorders. Hamstring tightness may contribute to an increase in patellofemoral joint reaction forces. Tight hamstrings increase knee flexion during running, thus increasing the PFJRF instance (see Fig. 5-29); increased peri-patellar soft tissue tension from quadriceps tightness may also produce higher PFJRF. Gastrocnemius-soleus inflexibility causes compensatory pronation of the foot, resulting in increased tibial rotation and subsequent additional patellofemoral stress. Iliotibial band tightness can contribute to lateral tracking of the patella.

Some special maneuvers used for determining tightness of these structures are described on pp. 246 and 247.

The *passive patellar tilt* test is performed with the knee extended and the quadriceps relaxed. The examiner lifts the lateral edge of

TABLE 5-5 **EMG Recordings of the VMO**

	Normal Subjects	Patients With Patellofemoral Pain
VMO:VL ratio	1:1	<1:1
Activity	VMO tonically active	VMO phasically active

the patella from the lateral femoral condyle (Fig. 5-34). An excessively tight lateral retinaculum is demonstrated by a neutral or negative angle to the horizontal. A preoperative negative passive patellar tilt (therefore excessive lateral tightness) correlates with a successful result after a lateral retinacular release in those who do not respond favorably to conservative measures.

The *patellar glide test* indicates medial or lateral retinacular tightness and/or integrity. With the knee flexed 10 to 30 degrees and the quadriceps relaxed, the patella is divided into longitudinal quadrants. The examiner attempts to displace the patella in a medial direction, then in a lateral direction using the index finger and thumb (Fig. 5-35). This determines lateral and medial parapatellar tightness, respectively. A medial glide of one quadrant is consistent with a tight lateral retinaculum and often correlates with a negative passive patellar tilt test. A medial glide of three to four quadrants suggests a hypermobile patella. A lateral glide of three quadrants is suggestive of an in-

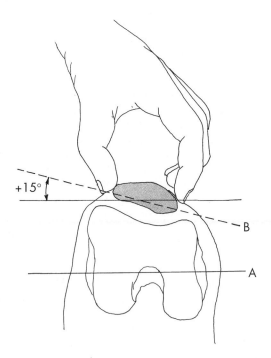

Figure 5-34 Passive patellar tilt test. An excessively tight lateral restraint (lateral retinaculum) is demonstrated by a neutral or negative angle to the horizontal. This test is performed with the knee extended and the quadriceps relaxed. (Redrawn from Kolowich P: Lateral release of the patella: indications and contraindication, *Am J Sports Med* 14(4):359, 1990.)

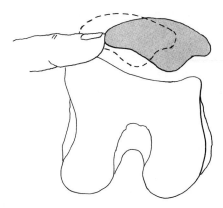

Figure 5-35 Patellar glide test is performed in 30 degrees of flexion. An attempt is made to displace the patella medially and then laterally to determine lateral and medial retinacular tightness, respectively. (Redrawn from Kolowich P: Lateral release of the patella: indications and contraindication, *Am J Sports Med* 14(4):359, 1990.)

competent medial restraint. A lateral glide of four quadrants (dislocatable patella) is obviously indicative of a deficient medial restraint.

Ober's test for iliotibial band tightness (see Fig. 5-21) is used to evaluate iliotibial band flexibility. It is performed by having the patient side-lying with the lower leg flexed 90 degrees at the knee for support and the pelvis stabilized. With the upper knee flexed at 90 degrees, the hip is brought from flexion/abduction to neutral (in line with the trunk) with neutral rotation and then is allowed to adduct. Both lower extremities are examined for comparison. The involved lower extremity exhibits iliotibial band tightness if the hip cannot adduct beyond neutral as far as the uninvolved side.

Endurance
Most authors encourage endurance training in patients with patellofemoral disorder. Bicycling and swimming are used most often because of their low-impact force on the lower extremities. Ericson and Nisell advocate a high saddle position during bicycling to minimize PFJRF during cycling. Stair-climber machines can be used to increase endurance, but caution must be taken to avoid increasing symptoms with this method.

Functional Training
The trend of therapeutic exercises for patellofemoral disorder has been toward more functionally oriented activities per-

formed with good VMO control. Several authors advocate a progressive running-agility-drill program that moves from basic to more advanced activities. They emphasize the use of electromyogram (EMG) biofeedback to facilitate VMO control of the patella during functional activities. Again, the absence of patellofemoral symptoms is a key guide to progression.

Rest

Because many forms of patellofemoral disorders are caused by overuse, various levels of rest are recommended as part of the treatment algorithm. Relative rest from activity is obtained by modifying the offending activity or selecting other activities to decrease symptoms. Absolute or complete rest is rarely recommended unless conservative treatment fails.

Medication

NSAIDs are often used unless contraindicated. Iontophoresis has had some success. Steroid injection is discouraged because of resultant articular cartilage degradation and possible tendon rupture.

External Support

Several methods have been reported for externally supporting the patella in patients with patellofemoral disorder. Many authors advocate a dynamic patellar stabilizing brace devised by Palumbo. McConnell has designed specific taping procedures to correct faulty patellar posture (see the following section). We have found taping to be helpful, especially when used during the transitional period required for the patient to strengthen the VMO. Taping increases effective quadriceps strength by decreasing pain and VMO inhibition. The actual VMO:vastus lateralis ratio is reported to be improved with patellofemoral taping. McConnell reports that taping applied after evaluation of patellar posture temporarily corrects abnormal tilt, glide, and rotation of the patella, facilitating normal patellar tracking in a pain-free manner. The patient can be taught to do the taping.

McConnell Taping Techniques for Patellofemoral Pain

- Clean, shave, spray with skin prep, and let dry.
- Cover the knee with 4-inch cover roll from midline lateral, over the patella, to under the medial hamstring group. Do not pull the tape tight.
- Outline the patella for better taping orientation. Mark into four quadrants and label.
- Place 6-inch brown Leukotape P over proximal/medial quadrant and apply pressure with the same-side thumb while pull-

ing the tape with opposite-side hand, medial, as tight as possible. This is known as **tilt component** (Fig. 5-36, *A*).
- Place 6″ Leukotape P over the proximal/lateral quadrant and, while pulling up on the medial thigh with the same-side hand, pull tape medial with opposite-side hand, again, as tight as possible to the underside of the knee. This is the **glide component** (Fig. 5-36, *B*).
- Place 3-inch tape over distal/medial quadrant, and turn the patella medial to correct external rotation of the inferior pole. Place the tape over the existing tape medial without pulling too tight. There should be no increased inferior pressure on the patella.
- Patient should then perform a **step test** (Fig. 5-36, *D*) to ensure the tape is correcting the patella orientation and that there is no increase in pain with tape. The **tilt component** is performed first, then a step test is applied. The **glide component** (if no improvement) is followed by a step test. If still painful, the **rotation component** is applied (Fig. 5-36, *C*), followed by a step test.
- Patients generally tape every day for 6 weeks, placing the tape on first thing in the morning and removing it last thing before bed. Taping duration may be decreased to less time if there is a problem tolerating the tape. The tape should at least be worn during any physical activity.
- The tape must be removed during sleep to allow the skin sufficient time to recover.
- Tape should be removed very slowly. Pulling on the tape will irritate the skin and prevent future taping. Medisolve or Desolvit can be used to aid in tape removal.

Modalities
Because joint distension (effusion) often inhibits quadriceps muscle function (especially VMO), reduction of swelling is important to establish VMO control. Ice has been the most successful modality to reduce pain, inflammation, and swelling. Electrical muscle stimulation (EMS) has shown no significant strength gains over exercise control groups in normal subjects; however, in patients with ACL reconstructions, EMS groups showed improved strength compared with exercise-only groups.

Biomechanics
Excessive pronation of the foot results in compensatory internal tibial rotation, which can increase patellofemoral stress. Abnormal mechanics should be corrected with foot orthotics when appropriate (see *Clinical Orthopaedic Rehabilitation*). The patient should be evaluated for possible imbalances in strength and flexibility around the hip that may be causing excessive patellofemoral stress due to faulty patterns of movement during functional activities.

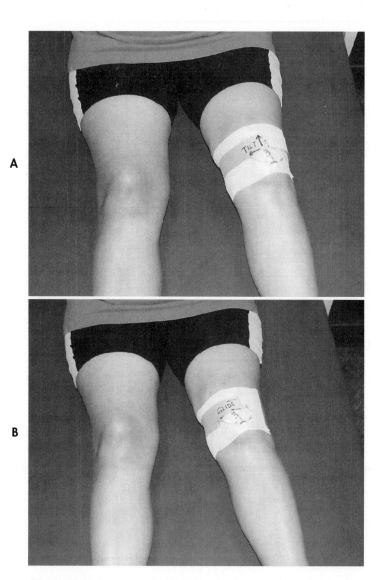

Figure 5-36 McConnell taping is based on an assessment of patellar position and maltracking. Three abnormal patellar orientations are examined: **A,** Tilt component, **B,** Glide component.

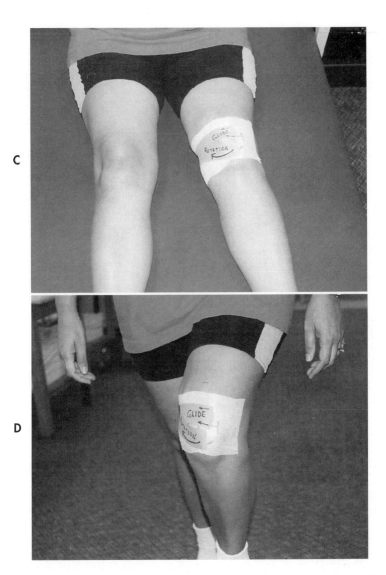

Figure 5-36, cont'd C, Rotation component. D, A step-test is performed between each to determine if this lessens the pain.

REHABILITATION PROTOCOL

Patellofemoral (Anterior) Knee Pain ROSS AND BROTZMAN

- May begin with modalities such as cold pack with interferential electrical stimulation (IF-ES) before exercises to decrease pain and swelling. May also require iontophoresis if tendonitis or reactive plicia is present.
- Perform all exercises with biofeedback over the VMO to ensure proper contraction and increase proprioception of the VMO.
- Patients begin with McConnell taping on the first visit. If the taping is tolerated well, they are instructed in self-taping on the second visit. The patient should be pain-free in the tape before initiating the exercise program.
- The patient is then instructed in open chain-table exercises on the first day. These include QS, straight leg raises, SAQ, hip adduction, flexion, extension and abduction, ankle plantar, and dorsiflexion as well as stretching the quadriceps, hamstrings, tensor, and gastrocnemius. Avoid hamstring stretching if the patient has recurvatum.

- If the patient is pain free with the open-chain exercises, begin closed-chain exercises. These include wall slides, lunges, lateral step-ups, balance board, heel raises, stool laps, hip adduction/SQ in standing, and leg presses.
- If the patient remains pain free with all the above exercises, begin stair-stepper, Fitter, stationary bicycle, and/or Versiclimber for general conditioning and endurance. The patient again receives a cold pack after exercise.
- Exercises are generally performed 3 to 4 times a week with a day's rest for muscle recovery. Repetitions are generally 3 to 4 sets of 10, with increasing resistance as tolerated.
- Allow return to full physical activity while taped if patient is pain free. Perform taping/exercises for approximately 6 weeks. At that time, discontinue the taping and continue the exercises as needed.

JUMPER'S KNEE

Rehabilitation Rationale

Jumper's knee was first described by Blazina et al. as tendonitis of the patellar tendon or quadriceps tendon at the inferior or superior pole of the patella, respectively. This definition was later broadened to include pathologic conditions at the bone-tendon junction of the patellar tendon on the tibial tuberosity (Fig. 5-37). Repetitive microtrauma results from the frequent use of the extensor mechanism in certain sports, such asvolleyball, basketball, track and field (high jumpers, long jumpers, sprinters, runners), and soccer. In adolescents, the same activities and repetitive microtrauma give rise to Osgood-Schlatter or Sinding-Larsen-Johansson diseases (Fig. 5-38).

Jumper's knee represents insertional tendinopathies of the quadriceps and patellar tendons. Patellar tendonitis is the most frequent tendonitis of the knee. It is localized at the lower pole of the patella and most often occurs in patients between the ages of 20 and 40 years. Quadriceps tendonitis is localized at the upper pole of the patella and is more frequent in patients older than 40 years of age.

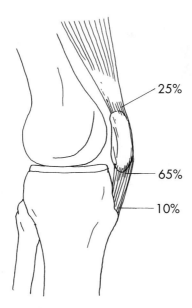

Figure 5-37 Location of pain in jumper's knee.

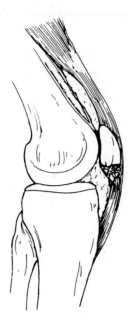

Figure 5-38 Sinding-Larsen-Johansson disease is an osteochondritis of the inferior pole of the patella in the skeletally immature. Conservative treatment leads to healing in 3 to 12 months. (From Colosimo A: *Orthop Rev* 19[2]:139, 1990.)

Differential Diagnosis of Jumper's Knee
- Bursitis
  Suprapatellar
  Prepatellar
  Subcutaneous
  Deep infrapatellar
- Patellofemoral arthrosis and chondromalacia
- Fat pad inflammation (Hoffa's disease)
- Meniscal pathology
- Synovial infrapatellar plica
- Osgood-Schlatter and Sinding-Larsen-Johansson diseases (skeletally immature patients)

REHABILITATION PROTOCOL

Prevention of Jumper's Knee DAVID

- Ensure warm-up of the entire body (5 minutes): Bicycle or upper body machine at low intensity or brisk walking
- Perform stretching (15 minutes):
  Quadriceps femoris
  Hamstrings
  Adductors
  Calf
  Iliotibial band
- Exercise:
  Rope jumping (5 minutes)
  Concentric/eccentric quadriceps exercise
  Curwin and Stanish's stop-and-drop program:
  Eccentric exercise program that places maximal stress on the tendon in an effort to increase its strength
  Patient drops to a semisquatting position, controlling the fall with an eccentric contraction

Drop is progressed by increasing the speed of descent until the patient is able to suddenly stop the freely falling body weight using the quadriceps eccentrically
  Plyometric exercises
  - Apply ice (15 to 20 minutes).
  - Repeat stretching.
  - Education:
  Frequency of training (reduction in activity when indicated)
  Type of playing surface (avoid hard playing surface)
  Proper shoe type and fit, orthotics if necessary
  Elastic knee supports, McConnell infrapatellar taping, or braces are utilized during training and games; we often use the patellar Aircast
  The reported mechanism of the patellar Aircast brace is compression of the tendon insertion of the patella and stabilization of the patella; during flexion of the knee the compression increases, decreasing the tensile stress and contributing to pain relief

REHABILITATION PROTOCOL

Symptomatic, Acute Jumper's Knee

REST

- As with other problems, a decrease in activity is indicated.
- The amount of inactivity depends on the severity of the injury and individual circumstances (recreational versus professional athlete).
- Cast immobilization is contraindicated. Immobilization results in muscle atrophy and weakened tendon, with recurrence likely when the now-weakened tendon is subjected to high tensile forces.

MEDICATION

- NSAIDs contribute to the conservative treatment of jumper's knee.

BRACING

- Avoid corticosteroid injections because of potential danger of tendon rupture.
- May use iontophoresis.
- Apply patellar Air cast or McConnell infrapatellar taping.

EXERCISE

- Use the same exercise program as outlined for anterior knee pain (Ross and Brotzman Protocol p. 252).

MODALITIES

- May use moist heat massage, ultrasound, phonophoresis, iontophoresis, electrical stimulation, and ice to provide different therapeutic effects that may be of benefit to the patient.

REHABILITATION PROTOCOL

Symptomatic Osgood-Schlatter Disease FOX AND DEL PIZZO

Phase 1
1 to 5 days

- If acutely symptomatic with limp, immobilize until acute symptoms decrease.
- Prescribe oral antiinflammatories if needed to reduce inflammation and pain.
- Apply ice.
- Use crutches if needed.

Phase 2

- Remove from immobilization
- May use an infrapatellar strap or protective brace with inferior horseshoe pad.
- Try interferential electrical stimulation to decrease inflammation if desired (may use in phase 1 also).
- Continue ice or oral antiinflammatories to decrease inflammation.

- Perform straight leg raises.
- Perform resisted plantar flexion of ankle with tubing.
- Begin short arc extension exercises, progressing to 1- to 2-lb weight and advancing in 2-lb increments.
- Begin isotonic exercises for hip flexors, extensors, abductors, adductors, and muscles of the lower leg.
- Achieve full ROM.
- Walk in chest-high water, use water vest, or swim to maintain cardiovascular fitness, or use a bicycle if it does not cause pain.
- Perform stretching exercises for hip and knee muscles.

Continued

REHABILITATION PROTOCOL—cont'd

Symptomatic Osgood-Schlatter Disease   FOX AND DEL PIZZO

Phase 3
- Continue to brace and use ice if needed.
- Continue ROM exercises.
- Perform strengthening exercises for hip and knee flexors, extensors, abductors, and adductors; do 3 sets of 10 repetitions, each starting with 3- to 5-lb weights and increasing by 2 lbs when exercise is done easily for the 3 sets.
- Start isometric exercises 0 to 90 degrees and include eccentric exercises for quadriceps;

e.g. lift 5 lbs from 90 to 0 degrees knee flexion, then slowly lower weight from 0 to 90 degrees (i.e., eccentric quadriceps activity) as tolerated.

Phase 4
- Add jumping, hopping, stepping.
- Jump off 8-inch step, then jump back up, first slowly and then more rapidly.
- Sport-specific skills where appropriate

CHAPTER SIX

Foot and Ankle Rehabilitation

S. BRENT BROTZMAN, MD
JILL BRASEL, PT

Ankle Sprains

REHABILITATION RATIONALE AND BASIC PRINCIPLES

Anatomy

The lateral ankle ligament complex includes the anterior talofibular (ATF), calcaneofibular (CF), and posterior talofibular (PTF) ligaments. The CF and ATF ligaments are synergistic: when one is relaxed, the other is taut. With the ankle plantar flexed, the ATF is more vulnerable to inversion stress; with the ankle dorsiflexed, the CF assumes a more important role.

■ *Because most ankle sprains occur in plantar flexion, the ATF is the most frequently injured ligament in inversion injuries.*

Classification

Rehabilitation of lateral ankle sprains is based on classification of severity (Table 6-1).

Evaluation

The talar tilt test examination is designed to reveal incompetency of the CF ligament (Fig. 6-1). The anterior drawer examination measures the integrity of the ATF ligament (Fig. 6-2).

Stress radiographs, such as the talar tilt test (for CF ligament incompetence), the anterior drawer test (for ATF incompetence), and stress Broden views (for subtalar instability) have been found

TABLE 6-1 Classification of Ankle Sprain Severity

Grade	Damage
1	Mild stretching of the fibers within the ligament, but no laxity, little swelling or tenderness
2	Partial tear of the ATF and CF ligaments with mild laxity, mild-to-moderate instability, moderate pain and tenderness, and some loss of motion
3	Complete ruptures of the ATF and CF ligaments that cause an unstable joint, severe swelling, loss of function, and considerably abnormal motion (electromyogram [EMG] studies also document an 80% incidence of peroneal nerve damage in grade 3 sprains, supporting the concept that the lateral peroneal complex provides an inversion restraint)

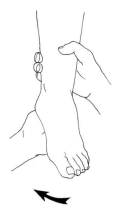

Figure 6-1 The talar tilt (inversion stress) test of the ankle.

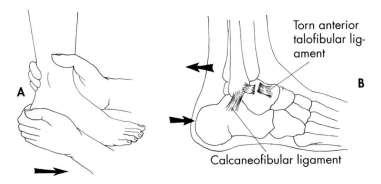

Figure 6-2 A, The anterior drawer test of the ankle. **B,** The integrity of the anterior talofibular ligament is assessed by the anterior drawer test. With complete disruption, the talus can be subluxed anteriorly beneath the tibial plafond.

to have questionable accuracy and reliability in the evaluation of ankle sprains because of variable parameters for "normal" (5 to 23 degrees talar tilt), and multiple variations among examiners (limb position, manual pressure, jigs).

Treatment

Most acute ankle sprains can be treated nonoperatively. Seventy-five percent to 100% of patients have good to excellent outcomes whether treated operatively or nonoperatively; those treated nonoperatively generally have fewer complications and more rapid recovery. Initial nonoperative, functional treatment is also supported by the very high success rate of reconstructive procedures for chronic ankle instability, such as those described by Bröstrom and Watson-Jones (Fig. 6-3). Failure of initial nonoperative, functional treatment still leaves the option of reconstruction with a high success rate.

Competitive athletes should first be treated functionally, with the realization that 10% to 20% may need elective secondary repair (Kannus and Renstrom). Exceptions include ballet dancers and members of the performing arts, whose activities involve "point" and "demipoint" positions (Fig. 6-4). Hamilton recommends open repair of acute grade 3 sprains in these athletes because of a high demand for healing without residual instability and the inadvisability of using a dancer's peroneus brevis for reconstruction of chronic instability.

Functional treatment (which includes only a short period of protection, early range of motion [ROM], and early weight bearing) has been clearly shown to provide the quickest recovery to full ROM and return to physical activity. It does not, however, compromise the late mechanical stability of the ankle more than any other mode of treatment (Kannus and Renstrom).

Van Moppens and Van den Hoogenband observed that at 9 weeks, patients who were immobilized in a cast or who underwent surgery had a higher rate of atrophy of the calf muscles than those who had functional treatment (18% and 22% versus 4%). However, at 6 months the difference was negligible. At 9 weeks,

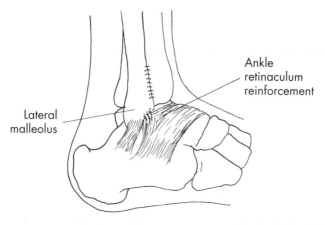

Ankle retinaculum reinforcement

Lateral malleolus

Figure 6-3 Modified Bröstrom ankle reconstruction.

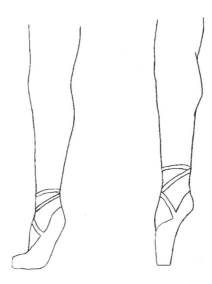

Figure 6-4 Demipointe and pointe in ballet.

68% of patients who had functional treatment had been restored to their preinjury levels of activity, compared with 7% of those who underwent operations and 13% of those who had only a cast. At 12 weeks, functional treatment still demonstrated a considerable advantage (81%, 36%, and 7%, respectively). Immobilization in a cast does have the benefits of providing a feeling of security for the patient, immediate painrelief, and less need for instruction, but muscle atrophy and stiffness are greater, and recovery is more prolonged. We use casts for noncompliant patients.

PREVENTATIVE MEASURES

Training Techniques
Two techniques often used by coaches and athletic trainers may help reduce the incidence of inversion ankle sprains:
- Peroneal muscle conditioning program before and during the season
- Teaching players to land with a relatively wide-based gait. This should place the foot a little more lateral to the falling center of gravity and make an inversion stress on the ankle less likely.

Prophylactic Ankle Taping
The efficacy of prophylactic ankle taping has been shown by numerous authors. In a study of 2562 basketball players, Garrick and

Requa found a lower incidence of ankle injuries for those who had prophylactic ankle taping. For patients with previous ligament injuries, ankle taping with high-top tennis shoes has been shown to be most effective in preventing reinjury (Lassiter). However, studies have shown that 12% to 50% of the supporting strength is lost in all taping methods after exercise, most occurring in the first few minutes (Rarick).

The open basket weave is one of the most common taping techniques used for acute ankle injuries (Fig. 6-5). The closed basket weave is often used after the risk of swelling has diminished (Fig. 6-6).

The best method of taping remains controversial. Frankeny et al. reported that the Hinton-Boswell method provided the greatest resistance to plantar flexion-inversion movements before and after exercise (Fig. 6-7). However, this method tapes the ankle in relaxed plantar flexion. Placement in dorsiflexion, where the ankle is more stable and extreme plantar flexion is less likely, appears to be a more logical choice. Others have found the basket-weave technique with a combination stirrup and heel lock to be the strongest method.

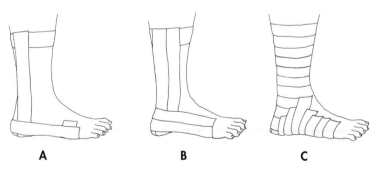

A   **B**   **C**

Figure 6-5 **A,** Open basket weave is performed immediately after injury because this technique allows for swelling. This taping provides compression and allows for swelling, but does *not* provide support. The player extends the lower third of the calf past the edge of the table. A heel pad is placed first. Two anchor strips are applied, then horizontal and vertical stirrups are added. **B,** Repeat the vertical stirrup, overlapping half of the previous strip. A second horizontal stirrup is then applied. **C,** Repeat the alternating vertical and horizontal stirrups. A 1-inch opening is left on the dorsum of the foot and leg. Overlap the previous strip by half. The ends are locked with long strips. (Redrawn from *Athletic training and sports medicine,* ed 2, Rosemont, Ill, 1991, AAOS.)

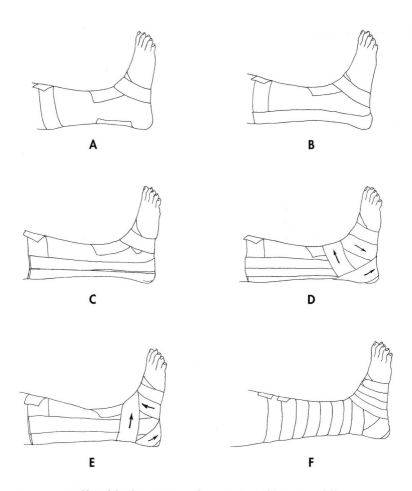

Figure 6-6 Closed basket-weave technique. **A,** Ankle taping following lateral inversion sprains: apply heel and lace pads, then apply two anchor strips. **B,** Apply stirrup strips, beginning on the medial part of the calf and passing under the heel. **C,** Continue applying strips up the lateral aspect of the leg; apply between three and six strips. **D,** Apply two to three heel locks in each direction. **E,** Apply figure-eight strips with force to cause slight foot eversion. **F,** Anchor tape components with fill-in strips, beginning at base stirrups and working up to proximal anchor. (Redrawn from *Athletic training and sports medicine,* ed 2, Rosemont, Ill, 1991, AAOS.)

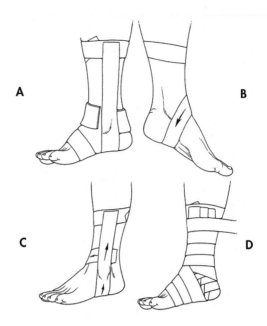

Figure 6-7 The Hinton-Boswell method of taping. **A,** Gauze pads, anchors, and stirrup applied. The anchors are placed at the musculotendinous junction of gastrocnemius and around the arch of the foot. The stirrup is placed medially to laterally, countering inversion forces. **B** and **C,** Two anchors and two stirrups are first applied with the ankle in dorsiflexion. Then, in relaxed plantar flexion, four figures of six are applied overlapping proximally to distally. **D,** Finally, a circular close is used to complete the wrap. (From Frankeny JR: *Clin J Sports Med* 3:1, 1993.)

Braces

Various ankle orthoses have been used in an effort to provide relative external support to the ankle without compromising ankle joint motion. In a study of collegiate football players, Rovere et al. found that lace-on stabilizers were associated with a lower incidence of ankle injury than was taping. However, Bunch found no significant difference in support between the two after 20 minutes of repeated inversion movements in the lab.

More recent designs include the use of semirigid plastics. Gross et al. demonstrated that these devices limited inversion-eversion motion significantly more than adhesive tape. Examples of these braces include the Aircast Sport Stirrup (Fig. 6-8) and the ALP (Donjoy). Currently there is little agreement in the literature about the effectiveness, support, and subjective comfort of various braces.

REHABILITATION

Ankle Sprains

The initial objective is to minimize swelling and inflammation. Cyriax explains that "the treatment of posttraumatic inflammation is based on the principle that the body's reaction to injury is excessive."

The RICE (rest, ice, compression wrap, elevation) regimen is used for acute injuries (see box, p. 268).

■ *Key recovery factors include protection, early motion and weight bearing, and rehabilitation.*

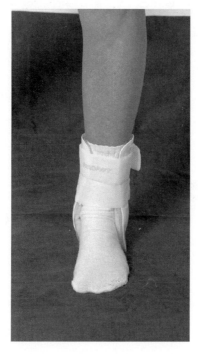

Figure 6-8 Aircast ankle brace.

RICE Regimen

Rest

Avoid activities that cause sharp pain.
Ensure the availability of crutches if the patient cannot walk without a limp.
Continue relative rest until the pain and swelling are negligible on weight bearing.

Ice

Ice provides local contraction of blood vessels so that blood flow is reduced to the injured area.
Reduction of swelling enhances healing.
Ice provides some pain relief.
Apply ice for 20 minutes initially every hour, then 3 to 4 times every 24 hours for 72 hours.

Compression

Various compressive dressings combined with ice decrease swelling in the acute inflammatory phase.

Elevation

Sims demonstrated with volumetric testing that elevated limbs have a significant decrease in volumetric displacement because the lymphatics have to work against decreased pressure to return excess fluid.
Guyton and Ganong demonstrated that as interstitial fluid and pressure increase past certain levels, a critical point is reached that causes collapse of lymphatic vessels.

REHABILITATION PROTOCOL

Acute Ankle Sprain MODIFIED JACKSON PROTOCOL

Jackson outlined a treatment regimen he used successfully for cadets at West Point. His program is divided into three phases. Using this regimen, disability averaged 8 days for mild sprains, 15 days for moderate sprains, and 19 days for severe sprains.

Phase 1
1 day

- Implement RICE regimen.
- Prescribe nonsteroidal antiinflammatory medications (NSAIDs).
- Use crutches if needed; allow weight bearing within limits of pain.

Phase 2—Restoration of Motion
Average times for phase 2 are as follows: grade 1 (3 days), grade 2 (4 days), grade 3 (5 to 9 days). (The reader must remember that this population of patients was 18-year-old cadets.)

2 to 12 days

- Begin ankle dorsiflexion and plantar flexion at patient's own pace, preceded by cool whirlpool and an intermittent Jobst pressure stocking (75 mm Hg).
- Use active ROM initially with no resistance to reestablish full ankle flexion and extension at the patient's own pace.
- Later, add rubber tubing resistance as tolerated.
- Begin heel cord stretches.
- Minimize dependent position of leg.
- Allow progressive weight bearing within the limits of pain.
- Initiate the following daily treatments for 1 hour each: 20 minutes cold whirlpool, 20 minutes intermittent pressure stocking, 20 minutes ROM exercises, plus ROM exercises at home.

Continued

REHABILITATION PROTOCOL—cont'd

Acute Ankle Sprain MODIFIED JACKSON PROTOCOL

Phase 2—Restoration of Motion—cont'd

2 to 12 days—cont'd

- Decrease the pressure stocking time as swelling diminishes.
- When patient is walking without a limp, has full painless ankle ROM, and is able to perform toe rise supporting body weight through the injured ankle, progress to phase 3.
- May begin swimming before weight bearing.
- Plantar flexion may be uncomfortable in water for grade 2 or grade 3 sprains with free-style because of resistance created by water.

Phase 3—Agility and Endurance

- Total body conditioning incorporated in each phase, but increased in phase 3.

- Perform strengthening exercises with emphasis on **peroneal tendons** and ankle dorsiflexors, the muscles responsible for actively resisting an inversion-plantar flexion injury.
- Isometric exercises:
  - Isometric strengthening against an immobile object or manual resistance:
    - Eversion (peroneals)—3 sets of 10
    - Dorsiflexion (dorsiflexors)—3 sets of 10
- Perform concentric and eccentric exercises with elastic band:
  - Concentric muscle contraction (muscle shortens) against the elastic band (Fig. 6-9, A).
  - Eccentric contraction (muscle lengthens) during the slow relaxation of the muscle as the elastic band overpowers the deliberately slowly relaxing muscle (Fig. 6-9, B).

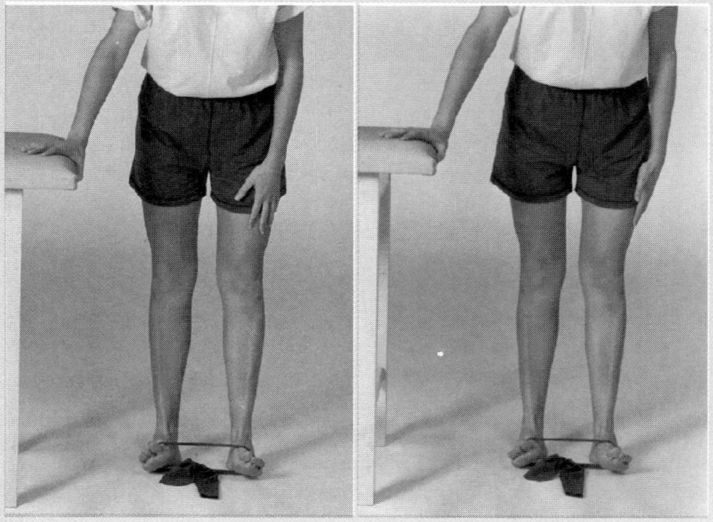

Figure 6-9 A, Concentric contraction (muscle shortens) outward against the band. **B,** Eccentric contraction (muscle lengthens) during slow relaxation of band.

Continued

REHABILITATION PROTOCOL—cont'd

Acute Ankle Sprain   MODIFIED JACKSON PROTOCOL

Phase 3—Agility and Endurance—cont'd

This slow muscle relaxation is emphasized to maximize the conditioning benefit of the eccentric contraction.

Eversion: 3 sets of 10

Dorsiflexion: 3 sets of 10

- Other exercises:

Toe raises (Fig. 6-10).

Step-ups: Patient approaches step from the side, lifts self using the injured extremity, and lands on the uninjured extremity. Patient then attempts to exercise facing the step, moving up and down in a forward/backward position (Fig. 6-11).

Skipping rope

Running on level ground

- Use proprioception board (balance board).
- Initiate BAPS (Biomechanic Ankle Proprioceptive System) (See Fig. 5-12): Trap and DeCarlo demonstrated a reduction in the number of recurrent ankle sprains after the use of proprioceptive/coordination training.

ACTIVITY PROGRESSION

The sequence for progression of activities is as follows:

1. Swimming, aquatic exercises
2. Walking; forward, retro
3. Jogging
4. Running
5. Figure-eights
6. Sport-specific agility drills

While resuming running, the patient should be instructed to run for 5 minutes and walk for several minutes, gradually increasing running time by 5-minute increments. If ankle pain occurs after 20 minutes, instruct the patient to drop back to 15 minutes until comfortable once more.

ORTHOTICS

- Occasionally we use an orthotic with a lateral heel wedge to place the hindfoot in hindfoot valgus in an effort to decrease the incidence of recurrent inversion injury and spraining.

Continued

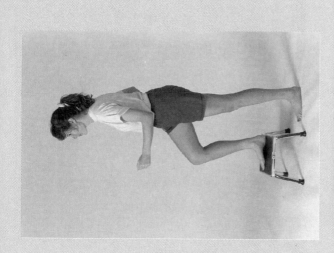

Figure 6-11 Step-ups.

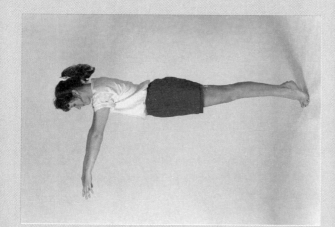

Figure 6-10 Toe raises.

REHABILITATION PROTOCOL—cont'd

Acute Ankle Sprain MODIFIED JACKSON PROTOCOL

Phase 3—Agility and Endurance—cont'd

ORTHOTICS—cont'd

- Patients with a pronated foot (pes planus) have been shown to have a reduced incidence of ankle sprains compared with those with a cavus foot. This fact also supports the use of a lateral heel wedge.

RETURN TO COMPETITION

- The athlete may return to competition when there is full muscular control of a painless joint with full ROM and no swelling.
- For 6 months after ankle sprain, athletes are advised to wear high-top shoes with taping or bracing (Aircast).
- Many authors believe taping, bracing, and high-top shoes also help by providing important sensory feedback.

BRACING FOR STABILIZATION OF THE ANKLE

Grade 1 injury
- We generally use an Aircast-type ankle splint in a high-top shoe for 3 to 6 weeks. We replace this with ankle taping and high-top shoes.

Grade 2 injury
- Same.

Grade 3 injury
- For compliant patients, we use a removable walking cast that affords added stability yet allows functional rehabilitation several times a day out of the walking cast. Weight bearing as tolerated (WBAT) with crutches is often required for the first several days. The removable cast may be replaced by an Aircast at 4 to 6 weeks.
- For noncompliant or very young patients, we often use a walking cast despite the increase in atrophy and added time required to return to competition.

REHABILITATION PROTOCOL

Severe (Grade 3) Ankle Sprains with Removable Walking Boot
MODIFIED LANE PROTOCOL

Requirements	• Adequate immobilization of the ankle • Accessibility for therapy exercises • Requires a compliant patient
Advantages	• Fewer complications from disuse and atrophy • Ease of application • Early return to sports with a stable ankle mortise
0 to 3 weeks	• Apply ice. • Elevate. • Wear walking boot (Fig. 6-12) at all times except during physical therapy. • Start immediate weight bearing as tolerated in boot (crutches may be required first week). • Perform daily physical therapy for first week, then 3 times per week for 2 weeks.	• May begin high-voltage galvanic stimulation (HVGS). • Use Jobst compression combined with elevation. • May use contrast baths (optional). • Perform isometric exercises in AFO.

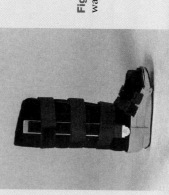

Figure 6-12 Removable walking boot.

Continued

REHABILITATION PROTOCOL—cont'd

Severe (Grade 3) Ankle Sprains with Removable Walking Boot
MODIFIED LANE PROTOCOL

3 to 5 weeks	• For first 3 weeks, maintain the ankle joint at 90 degrees at all times in therapy (using tape or other support). • Avoid eversion or inversion of the ankle.
	• Remove walking boot. • Change to Aircast-type brace and high-top tennis shoes. • Initiate gentle ROM and strengthening exercises: Isometric plantar flexion, dorsiflexion, inversion, eversion Rubber band exercises, same motions Step-ups Toe raises Calf stretches Stationary bicycle Swimming if tolerated without pain • Perform proprioception exercises with balance board at 4 to 5 weeks. • Avoid adduction and inversion ROM exercises for 6 weeks.
5 to 7 weeks	• Perform agility drills with Aircast or lace-up brace. • Perform proprioceptive exercises with balance board. • Continue rubber band eccentric strengthening exercises, concentrating on ankle eversion. • Perform agility drills: Figure-eights Backward running Cariocas
7 weeks	• Begin sports-related activities with taping or Aircast and high-top shoes. • Continue taping for 6 to 12 months. • Continue peroneal eversion rubber band exercises. • If ankle instability episodes recur despite good compliance, reevaluate exam and clinical situation.

REHABILITATION PROTOCOL

After Modified Broström Ankle Ligament Reconstruction
MODIFIED HAMILTON PROTOCOL

0 to 4 days		• Place ankle in anterior/posterior plaster splints in neutral dorsiflexion and discharge patient as non–weight bearing.
4 to 7 days		• When swelling has subsided, apply a short leg walking cast with the ankle at neutral. • Allow weight bearing as tolerated in cast.
4 weeks		• Remove cast. • Apply air splint (Aircast, etc.) for protection, to be worn for 6 to 8 weeks after surgery. • Begin gentle ROM exercises of ankle.

6 weeks
(Campbell Clinic modification)
		• Begin isometric peroneal strengthening exercises.
		• **Avoid** adduction and inversion until 6 weeks postoperatively.
		• Begin swimming.
		• Begin proprioception/balancing activities:
		  1. Unilateral balancing for timed intervals
		  2. Unilateral balancing with visual cues
		  3. Balancing on one leg and catching of #2 plyoball
		  4. Slide board, increasing distance
		  5. Fitter activity, catching ball

Continued

REHABILITATION PROTOCOL—cont'd

After Modified Broström Ankle Ligament Reconstruction
MODIFIED HAMILTON PROTOCOL

6 weeks (Campbell Clinic modification) —cont'd	6. Side-to-side bilateral hopping (progress to unilateral) 7. Front-to-back bilateral hopping (progress to unilateral) 8. Diagonal patterns, hopping 9. Minitramp jogging 10. Shuttle leg press and rebounding, bilateral and unilateral 11. Positive deceleration, ankle everters, Kin-Com • Complete rehabilitation of the peroneals is essential.	• Dancers should perform peroneal exercises in full plantar flexion, the position of function in these athletes (Fig. 6-13, A). • Early in rehabilitation, pool exercises may be beneficial (Fig. 6-13, B). • Dancers should perform plantar flexion/eversion exercises with a weighted belt (2 to 20 lbs).
8 to 12 weeks		• Patient can return to dancing or sports at 8 to 12 weeks after surgery if peroneal strength is normal.

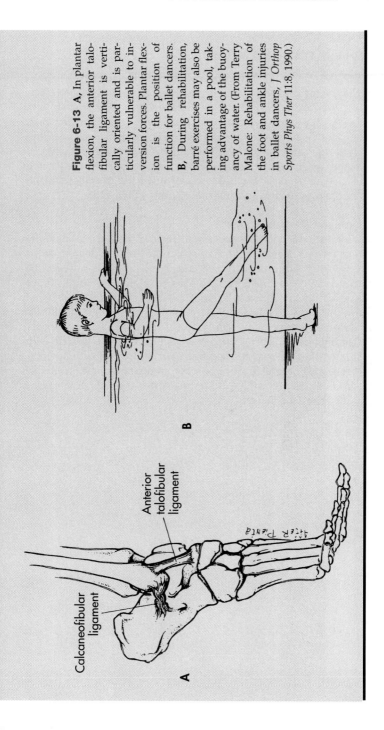

Figure 6-13 A, In plantar flexion, the anterior talofibular ligament is vertically oriented and is particularly vulnerable to inversion forces. Plantar flexion is the position of function for ballet dancers. **B,** During rehabilitation, barré exercises may also be performed in a pool, taking advantage of the buoyancy of water. (From Terry Malone: Rehabilitation of the foot and ankle injuries in ballet dancers, *J Orthop Sports Phys Ther* 11:8, 1990.)

Ankle Fractures

REHABILITATION RATIONALE

Weber classified ankle fractures into three types based on the level of the fibular fracture relative to the tibiotalar joint (plafond) (Fig. 6-14). Type A is distal to the tibiotalar joint; type B is even with the tibiotalar joint; and type C is proximal to the tibiotalar joint. This classification is helpful in making treatment decisions (operative versus nonoperative). The higher the fracture of the fibula, the more extensive the damage to the syndesmosis ligaments, and thus the more likely the ankle mortise will be unstable and require open reduction and internal fixation (Table 6-2).

Treatment Considerations

Anatomic reduction is necessary to restore the normal anatomy of this weight-bearing joint. Ramsey and Hamilton demonstrated that a 1-mm lateral shift of the talus in the mortise reduces the contact area of the ankle by 42%. This has significant implications for development of tibiotalar joint arthritis. Yablon et al. showed the talus follows the lateral malleolus deformity. Ankle stability is related to integrity of the syndesmosis and malleolar ligaments.

Undisplaced fractures with an intact mortise are treated with cast immobilization. Displaced fractures are treated with open reduction and internal fixation, unless an anatomic and stable reduction can be achieved with casting (often the reduction can be obtained, but not maintained).

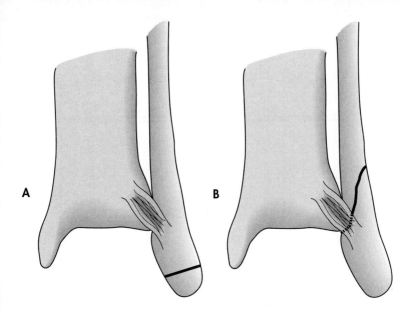

A

Weber A fracture
Fracture below the syndesmosis

B

Weber B
Fracture at the syndesmosis

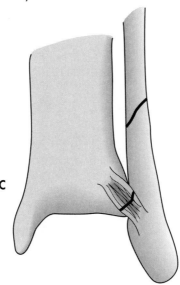

C

Weber C
Fracture above the syndesmosis
(unstable mortise)

Figure 6-14 A, Weber type A fracture: fracture below the syndesmosis.
B, Weber type B fracture: fracture at the syndesmosis. **C,** Weber type C
fracture: Fracture above the syndesmosis (unstable mortise).

TABLE 6-2 Types of Ankle Fractures

Weber Type	Description	Lauge-Hansen Equivalent (Foot Position at Time of Injury—Direction of Force)
A	Transverse avulsion fracture below level of plafond Syndesmosis intact Ankle mortise stable Typically does not require surgery	Supination—adduction
B	Spiral fracture beginning at the level of the plafond and extending proximally Interosseous ligament usually intact Anterior and posterior inferior tibiofibular ligaments may be torn, depending on the level of the fracture and severity of injury May or may not require surgery, depending on displacement, clinical picture	Supination—eversion
C	Fractured above the syndesmosis Syndesmosis torn, unstable ankle mortise Requires open reduction and internal fixation to stabilize ankle mortise	Pronation—eversion Pronation—abduction

Modified from Mann RA, Coughlin MJ: *Surgery of the foot and ankle*, ed 6, St. Louis, 1993, Mosby.

REHABILITATION PROTOCOL

After Stable Open Reduction and Internal Fixation of Bimalleolar or Trimalleolar Ankle Fracture

INDICATIONS
- Compliant patient
- Stable fixation

1 day
- Apply Jones-type dressing (well padded) with posterior splint and stirrup splint for 1 to 2 weeks; avoid equinus (neutral).
- Maintain maximal elevation for 48 to 72 hours.
- Ensure non–weight bearing with crutches.

and begin gentle, non–weight bearing active ROM exercises:
  Plantar flexion: 4 sets of 15 each day
  Dorsiflexion: 4 sets of 15 each day
  Straight leg raises (SLRs) and quadriceps sets for general lower extremity strengthening
- Perform gentle towel stretches (especially dorsiflexion) 2 to 3 times a day for ROM (Fig. 6-15).
- Taylor advocates use of a short leg cast with the distal portion of the front of the cast removed (to allow dorsiflexion). He then slips the cast downward so the ankle can be plantar flexed. We have encountered
  Continued

2 to 3 weeks
- Evaluate the wound.
- If wound is stable and fixation is stable, place highly compliant patients in a removable commercial cast (touchdown weight bearing)

REHABILITATION PROTOCOL—cont'd

After Stable Open Reduction and Internal Fixation of Bimalleolar or Trimalleolar Ankle Fracture

2 to 3 weeks —cont'd

problems with cast fit, rubbing, and abrasions, and we do not use this technique.

- Continue touchdown weight bearing with crutches for 6 weeks. If fixation is very stable, we allow partial weight bearing with crutches at 4 weeks, if this can be done without pain.

6 weeks

- Place patient in a removable commercial walking cast if not already in one and allow weight-bearing ambulation to tolerance for 2 to 4 weeks. Later replace with an Aircast-type ankle splint, to be worn until full ROM and strength are reestablished.

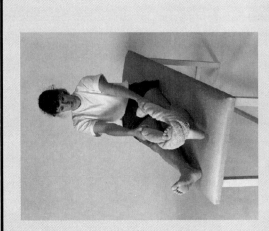

Figure 6-15 Towel stretches of calf.

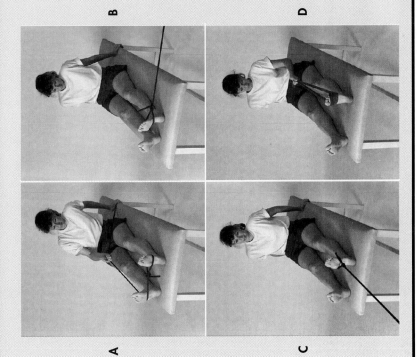

Figure 6-16 A, Resisted eversion of ankle. With tubing anchored around uninvolved foot, slowly turn involved foot outward (eversion). This exercise is the most important of this series. **B,** Resisted inversion. Inversion against Theraband. **C,** Resisted dorsiflexion of ankle. Anchor tubing on a stationary object. Pull foot toward body. **D,** Resisted plantar flexion of ankle. Place tubing around foot. Press foot down against tube into dorsiflexion.

Continued

REHABILITATION PROTOCOL—cont'd

After Stable Open Reduction and Internal Fixation of Bimalleolar or Trimalleolar Ankle Fracture

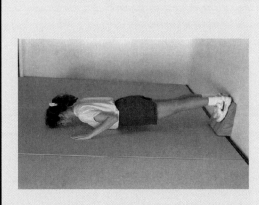

Figure 6-17 Incline board.

6 weeks—cont'd

- Remove the brace 4 to 5 times a day for therapy. Begin isometric strengthening exercises:
  - Dorsiflexion
  - Plantar flexion
  - Eversion
  - Inversion
- Initiate concomitant Theraband exercises (eccentric strengthening) at this time and progress through bands of incrementally harder resistance (Fig. 6-16).
- Begin stretching exercises for ROM:
  - Achilles tendon stretching
  - Runners' stretch
  - Incline board (Fig. 6-17)
  - Peroneal tendon stretching
  - Plantar-flexion stretching

| 6 weeks —cont'd | • Use joint mobilization if significant capsular tightness and stable fracture are present.
• Do proprioception activities: BAPS board or kinesthetic agility training (KAT) device
• Perform toe crawling with towel
• Perform closed-chain activities:
  Progression as tolerated—
  Wall slides
  Lunges
  Lunges with weight on shoulders
    Stair-climber | • Incorporate stationary bicycling to enhance ROM and aerobic conditioning.
• Use DOT drill.
• After acceptable ROM, proprioception, and strength have been restored, instruct patient on home exercises for progressive closed-chain strengthening and preathletic training drills (if relevant).
• Removal of syndesmosis screw if required. |

DELAYED REHABILITATION PROTOCOL

After Open Reduction and Internal Fixation of Bimalleolar or Trimalleolar Ankle Fracture

INDICATIONS	• Unstable fracture configuration, such as comminuted Weber type C fracture • Noncompliant patient		• Place in well-padded, short leg, non-weight-bearing cast at 1 to 2 weeks. • Maintain in cast for 6 to 7 weeks, non–or touchdown weight bearing. • Instruct in active ROM exercises of knee, straight leg raises.
1 day	• Apply Jones-type dressing (well padded) with posterior splint and stirrup for 2 to 3 days. • Maintain maximal elevation is for 48 to 72 hours. • Ensure non–weight bearing with crutches.	6 weeks	• Initiate exercises of previous protocol (see p. 283) when clinical union is evident.

Achilles Tendonitis and Peritendonitis
REHABILITATION RATIONALE AND BACKGROUND

Puddu et al. classified Achilles tendonitis into three types: pure peritendonitis, peritendonitis with tendonitis, and pure tendonitis. The *painful arc sign* is helpful in distinguishing peritendonitis from actual tendonitis. The foot is moved from dorsiflexion to plantar flexion (Fig. 6-18). In patients with peritendonitis, the tenderness and swelling *remain fixed* in reference to the malleoli (i.e., in the tendon sheath) as the foot goes from dorsiflexion to plantar flexion. In patients with tendonitis, the tenderness and swelling *move* with the tendon as the foot goes from dorsiflexion to plantar flexion. Magnetic resonance imaging (MRI) also may help to distinguish peritendonitis from tendonitis.

Anatomy

The blood supply to the tendon is via its investing mesotenon, with the richest supply emerging anteriorly (Schatzker). Lagergren and Lindholm found decreased vascularity in the Achilles tendon 2 to 6 cm above the insertion of the tendon.

The location of Achilles tendonitis is either at the insertion, in an area 2 to 6 cm proximal to the insertion (relative avascular zone), or at the musculotendinous junction ("tennis leg").

Etiology

Approximately 80% of patients with Achilles tendonitis are males. Clement et al. reported that 75% of Achilles tendonitis could be attributed to training errors. Multiple authors report functional overpronation as a common etiologic factor in Achilles tendon disorders (Fig. 6-19, *A*).

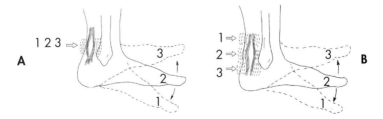

Figure 6-18 Painful arc sign. **A,** In peritendonitis, the tenderness remains in one position despite moving the foot from dorsiflexion to plantar flexion. **B,** In the case of partial tendon rupture or tendonitis, the point of tenderness *moves* as the foot goes from dorsiflexion to plantar flexion. (Redrawn from Williams JGP: *Sports Med* 3:114, 1986.)

Clement and Smart, through observations of slow-motion cinematography, determined that prolonged pronation causes tibial internal rotation, pulling the Achilles tendon medially. At push off, there is a resultant bowstring or "whipping" effect, pulling the tendon laterally (Fig. 6-19, B). This whipping action contributes to microtears and subsequent degeneration. These authors also describe conflicting rotatory forces imparted to the tibia by simultaneous pronation and knee extension, causing vascular impairment by blanching or "wringing out" of the vessels in the zone of relative tendon avascularity. This leads to subsequent degenerative changes (Fig. 6-20). Kvist also found markedly limited total passive subtalar joint mobility or ankle dorsiflexion limitation in 70% of athletes with insertional pain and in 58% of athletes with peritendonitis, compared with 44% of control athletes.

Achilles tendon overuse injuries can be best characterized as a spectrum of disease ranging from inflammation of the paratendinous tissue (paratendinitis), to structural degeneration of the tendon (tendonosis), and finally tendon rupture.

■ *The highest stress on the Achilles tendon during sports occurs during eccentric contraction of gastrocnemius and soleus complex; for example, pushing off the weight-bearing foot and simultaneously extending the knee, such as in uphill running. Thus, eccentric exercises should be used for rehabilitation of athletes who will undergo these stresses in their sports.*

Severe Achilles Tendonitis

Typically these patients have attempted to "run through" their pain and have had no success. The ankle is tender on palpation and the patient is unable to perform usual activity.

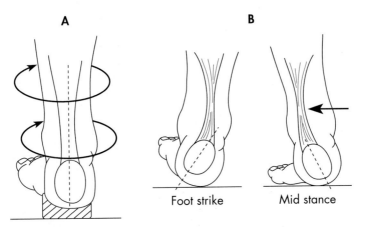

Figure 6-19 A, Correction of functional overpronation by medial rearfoot post minimizes potential for postulated vascular wringing. **B,** Whipping action of the Achilles tendon produced by overpronation. (From Clement D et al: *Am J Sports Med* 12(3):181, 1981.)

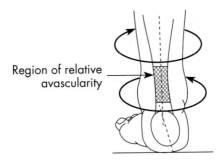

Figure 6-20 External tibial rotation produced by knee extension **(A)** conflicting with internal tibial rotation produced by prolonged pronation **(B).** This results in "wringing out" of vessels in the zone of relative avascularity. (From Clement et al: *Am J Sports Med* 12(3).

REHABILITATION PROTOCOL

Achilles Tendonitis in Running Athletes

CORRECTION OF TRAINING ERRORS	• Achilles tendonitis usually is related to a too rapid increase in frequency, duration, and intensity of training.
MODIFICATION OF RUNNING PROGRAM	• Stop hill running. • Decrease mileage significantly or initiate relative rest. • Increase cross-training in low-impact sports, such as swimming. • Stop interval training. • Change from hard to soft running surface. • Begin stretching program before and after exercise (Fig. 6-21); stress compliance. • Soften or cut out portion of a hard heel counter if causing posterior heel pain.

TREATMENT OF TENDONITIS	• Prescribe oral nonsteroidal antiinflammatories unless contraindicated.
	• Begin ice/cryotherapy:
	  Ice after exercise
	  Ice before exercise if soreness persists with exercise
	• Use iontophoresis.
	• Avoid cortisone injections (weakening and possible rupture of tendon).
	• Perform biomechanical foot and footwear correction if necessary (see *Clinical Orthopaedic Rehabilitation*).
	• Restore normal limb alignment if necessary.
	• Correct overpronation with biomechanical orthoses.

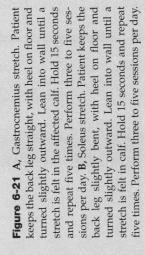

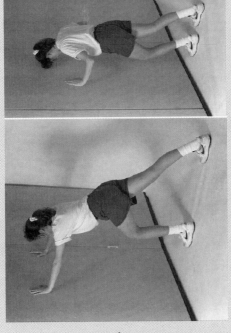

Figure 6-21 A, Gastrocnemius stretch. Patient keeps the back leg straight, with heel on floor and turned slightly outward. Lean into wall until a stretch is felt in the affected calf. Hold 15 seconds and repeat five times. Perform three to five sessions per day. **B,** Soleus stretch. Patient keeps the back leg slightly bent, with heel on floor and turned slightly outward. Lean into wall until a stretch is felt in calf. Hold 15 seconds and repeat five times. Perform three to five sessions per day.

Continued

REHABILITATION PROTOCOL—cont'd

Achilles Tendonitis in Running Athletes

| TREATMENT OF TENDONITIS —cont'd | • Some patients benefit from elevation of heel with small heel lift (¼ to ⅜ inch) to decrease excursion of tendon.
• Shoewear:
  Firm, close-fitting heel counters
  Wide heel base for rearfoot stability
  12 to 15 mm for heel wedge | Flexible sole to allow extension of metatarsophalangeal (MTP) joints at pushoff. (This will keep the lever arm from ankle to forefoot from being lengthened, which would otherwise increase the strain on the Achilles tendon.)
Avoid stiff-soled shoes; these increase the work of the muscle-tendon complex. |

REHABILITATION PROTOCOL

Mild Acute Achilles Tendonitis   MODIFIED DELEE PROTOCOL

INDICATIONS	• Onset of symptoms less than 1 to 2 weeks prior • Still able to perform activities (sports) despite pain
TREATMENT	• Prescribe oral nonsteroidal antiinflammatory medicine. • Ensure 2 weeks of rest from the aggravating activity. • Counsel on training and correct errors (p. 292). • Begin stretching regimen for gastrocnemius and soleus complex. • Begin eccentric exercise program 7 to 10 days after pain has subsided (see Table 6-3).

Eccentric Strengthening of Achilles Tendon   REYNOLDS

- Pain is the rate-limiting factor.
- Ensure that each level of progression is performed symptom-free before progressing to the next level.
- The progression should be slow to allow healing, rather than attempting to force a more rapid recovery and prolonging rehabilitation.
- Perform a toe raise on a 4-inch box or step. Both legs perform a toe raise. Once maximum plantar flexion is achieved, lift the uninvolved leg and lower the involved leg into dorsiflexion.
- Increase speed, sets, and weight to tolerance.
- Table 6-3 shows an example of an eccentric exercise program.
- Warm up–cool down before exercises:
    5- to 10-minute warmup
    Stretching: three 30-second stretches of the gastrocnemius and soleus.
- Stretch after the exercises and apply ice for 15 minutes with the ankle in a slightly dorsiflexed position
- Aquatic therapy is useful if the athlete is unable to bear full weight. Use a submersed brick to provide elevation. Submersion can begin at shoulder height and progress to waist height.
- A cycle ergometer (using lower extremities and moving upper extremities on the handle) is a useful cardiovascular adjunct.
- When the patient has reached phase 6, begin a walk/jog program. Perform frequent stops to stretch.
- Increase total walk/jog time to 1 hour. At this point, decrease jog duration and increase intensity.

TABLE 6-3 **Example of Toe-Raise Eccentric Exercise Program for Achilles Tendonitis (Reynolds)**

Phase	Sets/Reps	Speed	Weight	Frequency	Function*
1	3/10	Slow	Body	2×/day	ADLs sx-free
2	4/10	Mod	Body	2×/day	Mod walk up to 15 min sx-free
3	5/10	Fast	Body	2×/day	Fast walk up to 20 min sx-free
4	6/10	Slow	Body + 10 lbs	2×/day	Walk/jog 5 min/1 min sx-free up to 20 min
5	7/10	Mod	Body + 10 lbs	2×/day	Walk/jog 5 min/3 min sx-free up to 20 min
6	8/10	Fast	Body + 10 lbs	2×/day	Walk/jog 5 min/5 min sx-free up to 25 min

*Sx, symptom; min, minutes; mod, moderate.
From Reynolds J Orthop Sports Phys Ther 13(4):175, 1991.

REHABILITATION PROTOCOL

Severe Achilles Tendonitis BROTZMAN, RICHARDSON

- Stop running completely.
- Immobilize in a cast, commercial removable walking cast, or prefabricated AFO (depending on patient's compliance), to treat severe inflammation.
- Immobilization may range from 2 to 6 weeks, depending on severity of inflammation (usually around 3 weeks).
- May perform one-legged bicycling with uninvolved leg for cardiovascular fitness.
- Remove from cast when nontender to palpation.
- Initiate the following measures:
  - Gentle stretching exercises 2 to 3 times daily
  - Oral nonsteroidal antiinflammatory medications if not contraindicated

Cryotherapy

Slow, painless progression of activities:

1. Swimming
2. Bicycling
3. Walking
4. Light jogging
5. Eccentric exercises:
   - Aquatic exercises utilizing toe raises in pool
   - Toe raises with heel hanging over edge of stair
   - Progressively increase speed of heel drop
   - Rest if becomes symptomatic
6. Return to activity in graduated manner.

NOTE: This protocol takes into account the notoriously poor compliance of runners who are asked to quit running. We typically use a fiberglass cast that cannot be removed easily by the patient.

REHABILITATION PROTOCOL

Severe Achilles Tendonitis DELEE

- Stop the precipitating cause (running, etc.)
- Program of "modified rest":

  Stop precipating event (e.g., interval training, sprints)

  Allow patient to maintain aerobic fitness with alternative activities (e.g., swimming)

  Continue modified rest for 7 to 10 days after Achilles tendon pain has subsided

- Daily program of gastrocnemius and soleus stretching and strengthening exercises:

  Gastrocnemius and soleus stretches before and after exercises

- Initiate strengthening when pain has subsided:

  Toe raises with heel hanging over edge of an elevated object

  Move ankle through full ROM

  Begin eccentric exercise by progressively increasing the speed of the heel drop

- Correct functional components of foot malalignment with orthotic if needed.
- At 2 weeks after symptoms subside, begin a gradual return to the preinjury level of activity with a progressive, staged running program that increases intensity and duration.
- Return to sport is based on severity and duration of symptoms.

Turf Toe

REHABILITATION RATIONALE AND BASIC PRINCIPLES

The term turf toe includes a range of injuries to the capsuloligamentous complex of the first MTP joint. The mechanism of injury is hyperextension of the MTP joint (Fig. 6-22).

Predisposing factors include hard artificial playing surfaces (AstroTurf), soft-soled athletic shoes that allow hyperextension of the forefoot (Fig. 6-23), and occasionally a preexisting limited ROM of the first MTP joint.

Important diagnostic information includes the mechanism of injury, type of playing surface, type of shoe, exact location of pain, and the sensation of subluxation of the joint at the time of injury. Physical examination should note the presence or absence of ecchymosis and swelling around the MTP joint, ROM of the MTP, and localized tenderness of the sesamoids as well as of the dorsal or medial capsule.

In addition to the standard three views of the foot, medial and axial sesamoid views should be obtained.

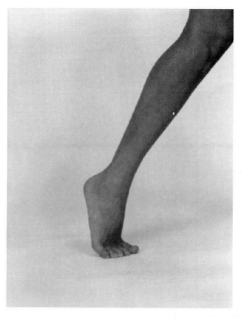

Figure 6-22 Hyperextension of first metatarsophalangeal joint.

PREVENTION OF INJURY

Stiffening of the forefoot of the shoe or use of a rigid orthosis may prevent turf toe. Several commercial orthoses are available that have a semirigid forefoot plate (steel spring plate) (Fig. 6-24). Normal active ROM of the first MTP is approximately 80 degrees, with 25 degrees of passive motion available (Fig. 6-25). At least 60 degrees of dorsiflexion is considered normal in barefoot walking. Stiff-soled shoe wear can restrict MTP joint dorsiflexion to 25 to 30 degrees without noticeably affecting gait (Clanton; Butler).

A stiff-soled shoe with a steel-plate insert is recommended to avoid reinjury by resisting hyperextension of the first MTP joint. After injury, a change to a wider or longer shoe may be necessary. Artificial turf shoes with more cleats of shorter length provide greater stability when bearing weight directly, as well as allowing sideward release with high shear forces (Sammarco).

Some authors advocate taping the first MTP joint in patients with turf toe to restrict dorsiflexion (Fig. 6-26). We have had limited success with this method, except when used with a stiff soled shoe for mild grade I injuries. This method loses significant support after the first 10 to 15 minutes of activity.

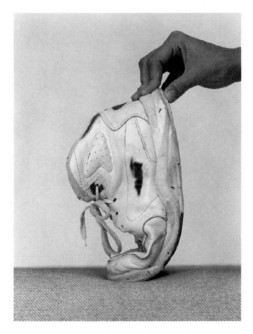

Figure 6-23 A shoe with a highly flexible insole offers little protection for a hyperextension injury.

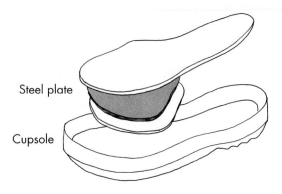

Steel plate

Cupsole

Figure 6-24 An exploded rendering of a shoe showing a plate of spring steel in the forefoot to prevent turf toe injuries.

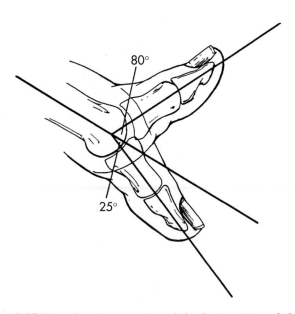

Figure 6-25 Normal active extension of the first metatarsophalangeal joint averages 80 degrees. Active plantar flexion averages 20 to 25 degrees. This excursion may decrease with advancing age. Also, 25 degrees of passive motion is available. (From Delee JC, Drez D Jr: *Orthopaedic sports medicine: principles and practice*, Philadelphia, 1994, WB Saunders.)

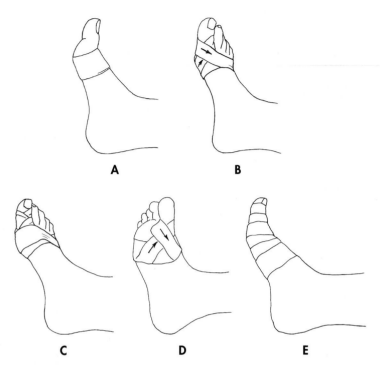

A   **B**

C   **D**   **E**

Figure 6-26 **A,** Great toe taping: begin procedure by placing an anchor around the forefoot, encircling the metatarsals. **B,** Apply half figure-eight taping at the first MTP joint and encircle the great toe. **C,** To prevent extension, repeat the figure-eight procedure two to three times. **D,** Begin figure-eight taping of the first MTP joint and encircle the great toe. **E,** Close in the toe and forefoot with overlapping strips applied distal to proximal. (Redrawn from *Athletic training and sports medicine.* AAOS 687, Fig. 43-33, *A-E.*)

Treatment

Both treatment and rehabilitation of turf toe are based on the severity of injury (types I through III), as indicated by the Clanton classification system (Table 6-4).

Patients may return to sports when the swelling of the MTP joint has resolved and may return to competition when full, painless ROM from 0 to 90 degrees has been obtained.

Typical time lost from sports for each type of injury is shown in Table 6-5.

TABLE 6-4 Clanton Classification of Turf Toe Injury and Treatment

Type	Objective Findings	Pathologic Condition	Treatment
I	No ecchymosis Minimal or no swelling Localized plantar or medial tenderness	Stretching of capsuloligamentous complex	Ice/elevation NSAIDs Rigid insole Continued participation in athletics
II	Diffuse tenderness Ecchymosis Pain, restriction of motion	Partial tear of capsuloligamentous complex	Same as type I Restriction of athletic activity for 7 to 145 days, depending on clinical course (see guidelines below under return to sports)
III	Severe tenderness to palpation Considerable ecchymosis and swelling Marked restriction of motion	Tear of capsuloligamentous complex Compression injury of articular surface	Same as type II Crutches and limited weight bearing If MTP dislocated, reduction and immobilization initially with cast Restriction of athletic activity (see guidelines on p. 305)

Modified from Clanton TO. In Brotzman SB, Graves SG: *Orthopaedic knowledge update: sports medicine*, Griffin LY, editor, Rosemont, Ill, 1993, AAOS.

GENERAL REHABILITATION PRINCIPLES

- Rehabilitation includes using early icing and elevation, NSAIDs, restriction from sports, and in some instances limited weight bearing.
- Begin active and passive ROM exercises of the MTP joint (both non–weight bearing and weight bearing) as soon as a decrease in symptoms allows (see protocol on p. 306).

TABLE 6-5 **Average Time Lost From Sports for Turf Toe Injury**

Type	Time Loss
I	Continued participation with rigid insole
II	1 day to 2 weeks
III	3 to 10 weeks

REHABILITATION PROTOCOL

Turf Toe (Non–Weight-Bearing Exercise Program)   SAMMARCO

Start by doing each exercise 10 times. Increase repetitions by 5 each day, up to a total of 30 repetitions. Do program 3 times daily. Exercise slowly and to the maximum stretch.

PULLING
EXERCISES

- Sit on floor with legs straight out in front. Place a towel around ball of foot. Grasp both ends of towel with hands, pulling foot toward knee. Stretch to the count of 5. Release.

- Same as above, except pull more with right hand to bring foot to right, then pull with left hand to bring foot to left.

- Repeat both with knee bent about 30 degrees.

FLEXING
EXERCISES

- Sit on floor with legs straight out in front. Flex foot upward, toward face, curling toes under at the same time, then point the foot downward, bringing toes up at the same time. The sequence is foot up, toes down, foot down, toes up.

- Sit on floor with legs straight out in front, placing both heel and ball of foot flat against a wall. Flex toes toward face. Hold to count of 5. Relax.

- Repeat both with knee bent about 30 degrees.

SLIDING
EXERCISES

- Sit in chair with knee bent and foot flat on floor under knee. Keeping heel and ball of foot on floor, raise toes. Keeping toes up, slide foot back a few inches, relax toes. Then raise toes again and slide foot back a few more inches. Keep raising the toes and sliding foot back until it is no longer possible to keep heel on floor while raising the toes.

SLIDING EXERCISES —cont'd

- From starting position, slide foot forward as far as possible, keeping both toes and heel in contact with floor. Keeping heel on floor and knee straight, flex foot up toward knee. Then point foot, pressing toes onto floor. Repeat, except keep toes curled while stretching and pointing foot.
- From starting position, "claw" the toes, inching foot forward as toes claw; then release. Separate toes between clawing. Inch out as far as possible, then slide back and start again.

PRESSING EXERCISE

- Sit in chair with knee bent and foot flat on floor under knee. Raise heel, keeping toes flat on floor; then press down again. Lean upper body forward for increased stretch.

ROLLING EXERCISES

- Sit in chair with knee bent and foot flat on the floor under knee. Turn inside edge of foot toward face (supinate), keeping outside edge on floor. Hold to the count of 5. Then flatten foot and bring outside edge toward face (pronate), keeping inside edge on floor, including big toe. Hold to count of 5. Do not let knee move during this exercise.
- From starting position, raise big toe, then next toe, progressing to little toe. Reverse, going from little toe to big toe.
- From starting position, slightly lift heel, putting weight on lateral borders of foot. Roll from little toe to big toe, then back through heel without letting heel touch the floor, making a complete circle around ball of foot. Repeat and reverse.

If edema and stiffness persist, contrast, whirlpool, and ultrasound with cold compression may be used as adjuncts. These modalities are aimed at decreasing edema, increasing motion, and mobilizing scar until symptoms subside.

Heel Pain

REHABILITATION RATIONALE

Heel pain is best classified by anatomic location (see box on p. 309).

This section discusses plantar fasciitis (inferior heel pain). Posterior heel pain is discussed in the section on Achilles tendonitis.

Anatomy and Pathomechanics

The plantar fascia is a dense, fibrous connective tissue structure originating from the medial tuberosity of the calcaneus. The fascia extends through the medial longitudinal arch into individual bundles and inserts into each proximal phalanx (Doxey).

The medial calcaneal nerve supplies sensation to the medial heel. The nerve to the abductor digiti minimi may be compressed by the intrinsic muscles of the foot. Some studies, such as those by Baxter and Thigpen, suggest that nerve entrapment (abductor digiti quinti) plays a role in inferior heel pain (Fig. 6-27).

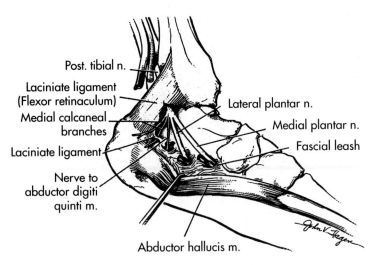

Post. tibial n.

Laciniate ligament (Flexor retinaculum)

Medial calcaneal branches

Laciniate ligament

Nerve to abductor digiti quinti m.

Lateral plantar n.

Medial plantar n.

Fascial leash

Abductor hallucis m.

Figure 6-27 Site of entrapment of the posterior tibial nerve and its branches, demonstrating possible entrapment beneath the laciniate ligament and at the point where the nerve passes through the fascia of the abductor hallucis muscle. (From Baxter DE, Thigpen CM: *Foot Ankle Int* 5(1):16, Copyright American Orthopaedic Foot and Ankle Society, 1984. From Delee JC, Drez D Jr: *Orthopedic sports medicine: principles and practice,* Philadelphia, 1994, WB Saunders.)

Differential Diagnosis of Heel Pain

Plantar (Inferior)
Plantar fasciitis/plantar fascia rupture
Calcaneal spur
Fat pad syndrome
Calcaneal periostitis
Compression of the nerve to the abductor digiti quinti

Medial
Tarsal tunnel syndrome
Medial calcaneal neuritis
Posterior tibial tendon disorders

Lateral
Lateral calcaneal neuritis
Peroneal tendon disorders

Posterior
Retrocalcaneal bursitis
Calcaneal apophysitis (skeletally immature)
Haglund's deformity
Calcaneal exostosis

Diffuse
Calcaneal stress fracture
Calcaneal fracture

Other
Systemic disorder (often bilateral)
Reiter's syndrome
Ankylosing spondylitis
Lupus
Gouty arthropathy
Pseudogout
Rheumatoid arthritis
Systemic lupus erythematosus

Modified from Doxey: *J Orthop Sports Phys Ther* 9(1):26, 1987.

The plantar fascia is an important static support for the longitudinal arch of the foot (Schepsis et al.). Strain on the longitudinal arch exerts its maximal pull on the plantar fascia, especially its origin on the medial process of the calcaneal tuberosity. The plantar fascia elongates with increased loads to act as a shock absorber, but its ability to elongate is limited (especially with decreasing elasticity common with age) (Noyes). Passive extension of the MTP joints pulls the plantar fascia distally and also increases the height of the arch of the foot.

Etiology
Inferior, subcalcaneal pain may well represent a spectrum of pathologic entities including plantar fasciitis, nerve entrapment of the abductor digiti quinti nerve, periostitis, and subcalcaneal bursitis.

Diagnosis
Bilateral plantar fasciitis symptoms require ruling out systemic disorders such as Reiter's syndrome, ankylosing spondylitis, gouty arthropathy, and systemic lupus erythematosus. A high index of suspicion for a systemic disorder should accompany bilateral heel pain in a young male aged 15 to 35 years.

Signs and Symptoms
The classic presentation of plantar fasciitis includes a gradual, insidious onset of inferomedial heel pain at the insertion of the plantar fascia. Pain is worse with rising in the morning or ambulation and may be exacerbated by climbing stairs or doing toe raises. Morning stiffness is also common.

Evaluation of patients with inferior heel pain includes the following:
- History and examination (Table 6-6)
- Biomechanical assessment of foot:
  Pronated or pes planus foot
  Cavus-type foot
  Assessment of fat pad (signs of atrophy)
  Presence of tight Achilles tendon
- Evaluation for possible training errors in runners (rapid mileage increase, running on steep hills, poor running shoes, improper techniques, etc.)
- Radiographic assessment with 45-degree oblique view and standard three views of foot
- Bone scan if recalcitrant pain (more than 6 weeks after treatment initiated) or suspected stress fracture from history

- Rheumatologic workup for patients with suspected underlying systemic process (patients with bilateral heel pain, recalcitrant symptoms, associated sacroiliac joint or multiple joint pain)
- EMG studies if clinical suspicion of nerve entrapment

TABLE 6-6 **Anatomic Palpatory Signs of Heel Pain Syndromes**

Diagnosis	Anatomic location of pain
Plantar fasciitis	Origin of plantar aponeurosis at medial calcaneal tubercle
Fat pad syndrome	Plantar fat pad (bottom and sides)
Calcaneal periostitis	Diffuse plantar and medial/lateral calcaneal borders
Posterior tibial tendon disorders	Over the medial midtarsal area at the navicular, which may radiate proximally behind the medial malleolus
Peroneal tendon disorders	Lateral calcaneus and peroneal tubercle
Tarsal tunnel syndrome	Diffuse plantar foot that may radiate distally with tingling, burning, and numbness
Medial calcaneal neuritis	Well localized to the anterior half of the medial plantar heel pad and medial side of heel; does not radiate into distal foot
Lateral calcaneal neuritis	Heel pain that radiates laterally, more poorly localized
Calcaneal stress fracture	Diffuse pain over entire calcaneus
Calcaneal apophysitis	Generalized over posterior heel, especially the sides
Generalized arthritis	Poorly localized but generally over the entire heel pad

From Doxey GE: *J Orthop Sports Phys Ther* 9(1):30, 1987.

REHABILITATION PROTOCOL

Plantar Fasciitis

Plantar Fascia Stretching

- To stretch the plantar fascia the patient sits with the knees bent and feet flat on floor. The tops of the toes are gently bent up with the hand.
- With the ankle dorsiflexed, pull the toes back toward the ankle. Hold the stretch in a sustained fashion for 10 seconds, repeating 10 times a day. The stretch should be felt in the plantar fascia (Fig. 6-28).

Achilles Stretching

- Runner's stretch
- Incline board

Steroid Injections

- Patients often receive good response from injection of steroid and long-acting anesthetic into area of plantar fascia insertion.
- We do not use more than 2 to 3 injections over the initial 2 to 4 weeks.

- The possible risks of injection must be discussed with the patient and possible harmful long-term sequelae weighed against short-term benefits:
  Possible plantar fascia rupture with subsequent loss of medial longitudinal arch
  Fat pad atrophy
  Allergic reaction to medication
  Low risk of infection
  Fairly painful injection

Heel Inserts

- Soft, spongy bilateral heel cups (e.g., Viscoheels) or soft, semirigid orthotic if biomechanical correction needed.

Special Treatment Considerations for Runners With Plantar Fasciitis

- Maintain relative rest until asymptomatic.

Special Treatment Considerations for Runners With Plantar Fasciitis—cont'd

- James et al. recommend a 6-week timetable, starting with jogging a 7.5- to 8-minute-pace per mile 15 minutes a day for the first week back. Five minutes are added to the daily schedule until 40 minutes of painless nonstop running is achieved (De Maio and James).

- Other running modifications include decreasing velocity, shortening stride length, and decreasing heel contact.

- Train on soft surfaces (such as grass) to diminish impact.

- Training shoes should have the following:
  A firm heel counter to control the hindfoot
  A well-molded Achilles pad
  A beveled and flared heel to help control heel stability
  A soft cushion with the heel 12 to 15 mm higher than the sole
  Sole of the shoe under the forefoot with significant midsole cushion, but flexible over the metatarsal heads.

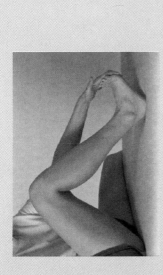

Figure 6-28 To stretch the plantar fascia, the patient sits with the knees bent and feet flat on floor. The tops of the toes are gently bent upward with the hand. Plantar fascia stretch. With the ankle dorsiflexed, pull the toes back toward the ankle. Hold the stretch in a sustained fashion for 10 seconds, repeating 10 times a day. The stretch should be felt in the plantar fascia.

REHABILITATION PROTOCOL

Evaluation-Based Rehabilitation Protocol for Plantar Fasciitis
MODIFIED DE MAIO AND DREZ PROTOCOL

	Weeks 1 to 4	Week 4 to 8 of Treatment	Week 8 to 12 of Treatment
Evaluation	• Confirm fascial origin of pain. • Evaluate for contributing factors: Overuse/training errors Biomechanics of foot (planus) Status of Achilles tendon (tight) Shoes (cushioning, appropriate fit) Body habitus X-ray Rule out inflammatory arthritis, nerve entrapment, stress fracture (see p. 311).	• Persistent pain • Confirm proper fit of orthotics. • Confirm diagnosis with review of history and physical exam • Review treatment regimen and assess patient's compliance	• Persistent pain • Medical workup • Bone scan Possible EMG if nerve entrapment is suspected. Rheumatoid profile lab and workup to rule out inflammatory arthritis Repeat x-rays

Treatment	• Use ice massage of insertion (antiinflammatory effect). • Prescribe NSAIDs unless contraindicated. • Modify shoe. • Fit soft, viscoelastic heel inserts. • Apply soft or semirigid orthotic if biomechanical correction needed. • Perform Achilles tendon and plantar fascia stretching (p. 313). • Reduce weight. • Modify activity (stop running for 6 weeks). • Maintain cardiovascular fitness (swimming, upper body exercise).	• Assess need for steroid injection (note risks). • Perform ice massage. • Taper NSAIDs. • Establish maintenance program. • Maintain fitness program. • With improvement, gradually return to previous activity. • Review training errors again with corrections.	• Use night splinting to decrease plantar flexion at night (Figure 6-29) • May use short leg walking cast for 4 to 6 weeks (or removable walking boot for highly compliant patient; removed only for bathing). • Use steroid injection (see risks). • In patients whose symptoms diminish, return to 4- to 8-week protocol. • Persistent symptoms for 6 months may require operative intervention
Goals	• Decrease inflammation • Relative rest • Correct underlying contributing factors • Increase flexibility	• Return to previous level of function • Prevent recurrence	• Confirm diagnosis

RUPTURE OF THE PLANTAR FASCIA

Rupture of the plantar fascia typically results in long-term loss of the medial arch of the foot. Treatment is nonoperative. Because unprotected weight bearing is painful in the acute phase, the patient is placed touchdown to weight bearing as tolerated with a removable walking cast and crutches. The acute phase often lasts 3 to 6 weeks. Protected weight bearing with a firm shoe and/or orthotic is begun after the acute phase subsides. Passive stretching exercises, local massage, and modalities are often begun after subsidence of acute pain. A custom-made semirigid or soft orthotic in subtalar neutral (see *Clinical Orthopaedic Rehabilitation*) is worn for support of the longitudinal arch of the foot.

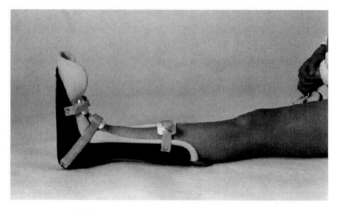

Figure 6-29 Position of night splint during patient use.

CHAPTER SEVEN

Rehabilitation After Total Joint Arthroplasty

S. BRENT BROTZMAN, MD
HUGH U. CAMERON, MD
MARYLYLE BOOLOS, PT

Total Hip Arthroplasty

REHABILITATION RATIONALE

The original primary indication for total hip arthroplasty of incapacitating pain in the patient older than 65 years of age, refractory to all medical and surgical therapy, has been expanded after the documented, remarkable success of total hip arthroplasty (Fig. 7-1) in a variety of disorders (see boxes).

GOALS OF REHABILITATION PROGRAM AFTER TOTAL HIP ARTHROPLASTY

- Guard against dislocation of the implant.
- Gain functional strength.
- Strengthen hip and knee musculature.

Disorders of the Hip Joint for Which Total Hip Arthroplasty May Be Indicated

Arthritis
  Rheumatoid
  Juvenile rheumatoid
    (Still's disease)
  Pyogenic
Ankylosing spondylitis
Avascular necrosis
  Postfracture or dislocation
  Idiopathic
Bone tumor
Cassion disease
Degenerative joint disease
  Osteoarthritis
Developmental dysplasia
  of the hip
Failed hip reconstruction
  Cup arthroplasty
  Femoral head prosthesis
  Girdlestone procedure
  Resurfacing arthroplasty
  Total hip replacement

Fracture or dislocation
  Acetabulum
  Proximal femur
Fusion or pseudarthrosis of
  hip
Gaucher's disease
Hemoglobinopathies
  (sickle cell disease)
Hemophilia
Hereditary disorders
Legg-Calvé-Perthes disease
  (LCPD)
Osteomyelitis (remote, not
  active)
  Hematogenous
  Postoperative
Osteotomy
Renal disease
  Cortisone induced
  Alcoholism
Slipped capital femoral
  epiphysis
Tuberculosis

Contraindications to Total Hip Arthroplasty

Absolute Contraindications

1. Active infection in the joint, unless carrying out a revision either as an immediate exchange or an interval procedure
2. Systemic infection or sepsis
3. Neuropathic joint
4. Malignant tumors that do not allow adequate fixation of the components

Relative Contraindications

1. Localized infection, especially bladder, skin, chest, or other local regions
2. Absent or relative insufficiency of the abductor musculature
3. Progressive neurologic deficit
4. Any process rapidly destroying bone
5. Patients requiring extensive dental or urologic procedures, such as transurethral resection of the prostate, should have this performed before total joint replacement

- Prevent bed-rest hazards (e.g., thrombophlebitis, pulmonary embolism, decubiti, pneumonia).
- Teach independent transfers and ambulation with assistive devices.
- Obtain pain-free range of motion (ROM) within precaution limits.

■ *Rehabilitation considerations in cemented and cementless techniques*
  - *Cemented total hip*
    Weight bearing to tolerance (WBTT) with walker immediately after surgery
  - *Noncemented total hip*
    Touchdown weight bearing (TDWB) for 6 to 8 weeks with walker. Some authors prefer partial weight bearing (PWB) of 60 to 80 lbs.

Most surgeons treat cemented and cementless hip devices quite differently. The cement is as strong as it is ever going to be within 15 minutes of insertion. Some surgeons believe that some weight-bearing protection should be provided until the bone at the interface with the cement, which has been damaged by mechanical or thermal trauma, has reconstituted with the development of a periimplant bone plate. This phenomenon takes about 6 weeks. Most surgeons, however, believe that the initial stability obtained with cement is adequate to allow immediate, full, unprotected weight bearing.

With noncemented hip prostheses the initial fixation is press fit. Maximum implant fixation is unlikely to be achieved until some tissue on-growth or in-growth into the implant has been established. Whereas fixation by 6 weeks is usually adequate, maximum stability is probably not achieved until approximately 6 months. For these reasons many surgeons advocate non–weight bearing or toe-touch weight bearing for the first 6 weeks. Some believe that the initial stability achieved is adequate to allow weight bearing as tolerated.

It must be remembered that straight leg raising can produce very large loads in the hip, and many surgeons prefer to avoid this, as well as side leg lifting in the lying position for the same time frame. Even vigorous isometric contractions of the hip abductors should be practiced with caution.

Initial rotational resistance of a noncemented hip may be low, and it may be preferable to protect the hip from large rotational forces for 6 weeks or so. The most common rotational load comes when arising from a seated position so that pushing off with the hands is strongly recommended.

Even after full weight bearing is established, it is essential that the patient continue to use a cane in the contralateral hand until limp stops. This helps to prevent or avoid the development of a Trendelenburg gait, which may be difficult to eradicate at a later date. In some very difficult revisions where implant or bone stability has been difficult to establish, the patient may be advised to continue to use a cane indefinitely. In general, when the patient gets up and walks away forgetting about the cane, it can safely be discarded.

The routines outlined here are general routines and may need to be tailored to specific patients. For example, weight bearing should be limited to touch if any osteotomy of the femur has been carried out. Osteotomies can be classified as alignment correction osteotomies, either angular or rotational; shortening osteotomies, such as calcar episiotomy or subtrochanteric shortening; and exposure osteotomies, such as a trochanteric osteotomy or slide, an extended trochanteric osteotomy or slide, or a window.

Expansion osteotomies allow the insertion of a larger prosthesis. Reduction osteotomies allow narrowing of the proximal femur. In these groups weight bearing should be delayed until some union is present. These patients should also avoid straight leg raising and side leg lifting until, in the opinion of the surgeon, it is safe to do so.

Treatment may also have to be adjusted because of inadequate initial fixation. In revision surgery a stable press fit of the acetabular component may be difficult to achieve, and multiple screw fixation may be required. Under those circumstances caution should be exercised in rehabilitation.

Treatment might also have to be adjusted because of stability. Revision to correct recurrent dislocations may require the use of an abduction brace to prevent adduction and flexion to more than 80 degrees for varying periods of up to 6 months. Similarly, significant leg shortening through the hip at the time of revision, with or without a constrained socket, should be protected for 3 to 6 months with an abduction brace until the soft tissues tighten up.

These considerations should be reviewed and integrated into a specific rehabilitation protocol tailored to the individual patient.

REHABILITATION PROTOCOL

Total Hip Arthroplasty

Preoperative

- Instruct on precautions for hip dislocation
- Transfer instructions:
  In and out of bed
  Chair.
  Depth-of-chair restrictions: avoid deep chairs. We also instruct patients to look at the ceiling as they sit down to minimize trunk flexion.
  Sitting: avoid crossing legs.
  Rising from chair: scoot to edge of the chair, then rise.
  Use of elevated commode seat: elevated seat is placed on commode at a slant, with higher part at the back, to aid in rising.
- Ambulation: instruct on use of anticipated assistive device (walker).
- Exercises: demonstrate day-1 exercises.

Postoperative

- Out of bed in stroke chair twice a day with assistance 1 or 2 days postoperative. Do **NOT** use a low chair.
- Begin ambulation with assistive device twice a day (walker) 1 or 2 days postoperatively with assistance from therapist.
  Cemented prosthesis: WBAT with walker for at least 6 weeks, then use a cane in the contralateral hand for 4 to 6 months.
  Cementless technique: TDWB with walker for 6 to 8 weeks (some authors recommend 12 weeks), then use a cane in the contralateral hand for 4 to 6 months. A wheelchair may be used for long distances with careful avoidance of excessive hip flexion of more than 80 degrees while in the wheelchair. Therapist must check to ensure that the foot rests are long enough. Place a triangular cushion in the chair, with the highest point posterior, to avoid excessive hip flexion.

Isometric Exercises (Review parameters, p. 320)

- Straight leg raises: tighten knee and lift leg off bed, keeping the knee straight. Flex the opposite knee to aid this exercise. Straight leg raises are more important after total knee arthroplasty than after total hip arthroplasty.
- Quadriceps sets: tighten quadriceps by pushing knee down and hold for a count of 4.
- Gluteal sets: squeeze buttocks together and hold for a count of 4.
- Ankle pumps: pump ankle up and down repeatedly.
- Isometric abduction with self-resistance while lying. Later, wrap a Theraband around the knees and perform abduction against the Theraband.
- 4-point exercise:
  Bend knee up while standing
  Straighten knee
  Bend knee back
  Return foot to starting position
- Hip abduction/adduction:
  Supine position: abduct (slide leg out to side) and back keeping toes pointed up. Make sure leg is not externally rotated or gluteus medius will not be strengthened.

Standing position: move leg out to side and back. Do not lean over the side.

Side-lying position: Lying on side, patient abducts the leg against gravity (Fig. 7-1). The patient should be turned 30 degrees toward prone to utilize the gluteus maximus and medius muscles. Most patients would otherwise tend to rotate toward the supine position, then abducting with the tensor fascia femoris.

■ *Cameron emphasizes that hip abductor strengthening is the most important single exercise that will allow the patient to return to ambulation without a limp. The type of surgical approach (e.g., trochanteric osteotomy) and implant fixation (cement) dictates the timing of initiating hip abduction exercises (see p. 320).*

Stretching Exercises

- 1 or 2 days postoperatively, begin daily Thomas stretch tests to avoid flexion contracture of the hip. Pull the uninvolved knee up to the chest while lying supine in bed. At the same time, push the involved leg into extension against the bed. The hip extension stretches the anterior capsule and hip flexors of the involved hip and aids with previous flexion contracture and avoidance of postoperative contracture. Perform this stretch 5 to 6 times per session, 6 times a day (Fig. 7-2).
  Continued

Total Hip Arthroplasty

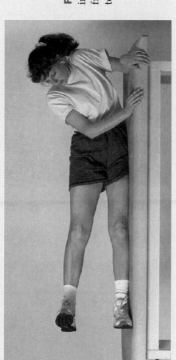

Figure 7-2 Thomas stretch tests: patient lying supine in bed, holding one knee flexed to chest, the other leg perfectly straight, pressing down on bed.

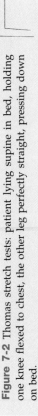

Figure 7-1 Side-lying hip abduction. Postoperatively, lying on side, lift involved extremity 8 to 10 inches away from floor. The patient should turn the body 30 degrees toward prone.

Stretching Exercises—cont'd

• May begin stationary exercise bicycling with a high seat 4 to 7 days postoperatively. To mount the bicycle, the patient stands facing the side of the bicycle and places one hand on the center of the handle bars and the other on the seat. Place the uninvolved leg over the bar and onto the floor so that the seat is straddled. Protect the involved leg from full weight bearing by pressure on the hands. With both hands on the handle bars and partial weight on the involved leg, place the uninvolved leg on the pedal. Stand on the uninvolved leg to sit on the seat. Then turn the pedals so that the involved leg can be placed on the pedal at the bottom of the arc.

Until successful completion of a full arc on the bicycle, the seat should be set as high as possible. Initially most patients find it easier to pedal backward until they can complete a revolution. The seat may be progressively lowered to increase hip flexion within safe parameters.

Initially the patient should ride the bicycle with minimal tension at 15 miles per hour, 2 to 4 times a day. We leave a stationary bicycle on the floor for use in the room. By 6 to 8 weeks, may increase the tension until fatigue occurs after approximately 10 to 15 minutes of riding.

• May also perform extension stretching of the anterior capsule (to avoid hip flexion contracture) by extending the involved leg while the uninvolved leg is mildly flexed at the hip and knee, supported by a walker (the therapist stabilizes the walker). Thrust the pelvis forward and the shoulders backward for a sustained stretch of the anterior capsule (Fig. 7-3).

• Observe and correct gait faults because many of these faults involve the patient's avoidance of stretching the anterior structures of the hip secondary to pain (p. 332).

Abduction Pillow

• Keep an abduction pillow between legs while in bed. *NOTE: many surgeons use a knee immobilizer on the ipsilateral knee during the first week to avoid possible prosthesis dislocation. Use the abduction pillow while asleep or resting in bed for 5 to 6 weeks; it may then be safely discontinued.*

Continued

REHABILITATION PROTOCOL—cont'd

Total Hip Arthroplasty

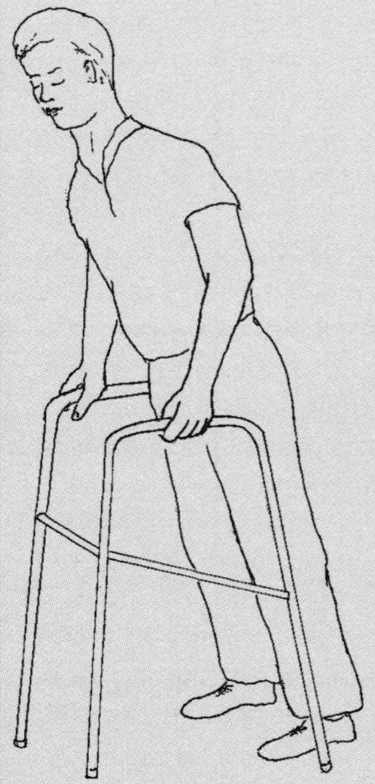

Bathroom Rehabilitation
- Permit bathroom privileges with assistance and elevated commode seat.
- Teach bathroom transfers when patient is ambulating 10 to 20 feet outside of room.
- Use elevated commode seat at all times.

Assistive Devices

Occupational therapist brings these and instructs patient on assistive activities of daily living (ADLs):

"Reacher" or "grabber" to help retrieve objects on the floor or assist with socks or stockings

Shoe horn and loosely fitting shoes or loafers

Transfers

Bed to chair:

Avoid leaning forward to get out of chair or off bed.

Slide hips forward first then come to standing.

Do not cross legs when pivoting from supine to bedside position.

Figure 7-3 Extension stretch while standing.

Precautions (Posterior Surgical Approach)

Do not lie on side that has undergone surgery until receiving clearance to do so from your surgeon.

Avoid crossing legs or internally rotating involved limb.

Keep abduction pillow between legs when in bed.

Keep legs separated when sitting.

Avoid low chairs that cause significant flexion of hip; knees should always be lower than hips.

Avoid low toilet (use elevated commode seat).

Avoid bending over to pick up objects (use a reacher); do not let hand pass knee.

Avoid sitting forward to pull up blankets (use a reacher).

Avoid leaning over to get out of chair; slide hips forward first, then come to standing.

Avoid standing with toes turned in.

Continued

Transfers—cont'd

Nurse or therapist assists until safe, secure transfers.

Bathroom:

Use elevated toilet seat with assistance.

Continue assistance until able to perform safe, secure transfers.

Transfer to Home

- Instruct patient to travel in the back seat of a 4-door sedan, sitting or reclining lengthwise across the seat, leaning on 1 to 2 pillows under head and shoulders.
- Instruct patient to travel in the back seat of a 4-door sedan, sitting or reclining lengthwise across the seat, leaning on 1 to 2 pillows under head and shoulders.
- Avoid sitting in conventional fashion (hip flexed more than 90 degrees) to avoid posterior dislocation in the event of a sudden stop.
- Urge those without a 4-door sedan to sit on 2 pillows with the seat reclined (minimize flexion of hip).
- Adhere to these principles for 6 weeks until soft tissue stabilization is achieved.
- May begin driving 6 weeks postoperatively.
- Review hip precautions and instructions with patient (see box).

REHABILITATION PROTOCOL—cont'd

Total Hip Arthroplasty

Posterior Hip Precautions

You have been instructed to **avoid:**

1. Crossing your legs or bringing them together—adduction.

2. Bringing knees too close to your chest—extreme hip flexion (you can bend until your hand gets to your knee).

3. Turning foot in toward other leg (internal rotation).

Listed below are several positions that could be part of your everyday activities. Remember to apply the above precautions.

1. When sitting, sit with knees comfortably apart.

2. Avoid sitting in low chairs and, especially, over-stuffed sofas or chairs.

3. Do not lie on the involved side until cleared by your doctor.

4. When lying on the uninvolved side always have a large pillow or two small pillows between your knees. Have the knees in a slightly bent position.

5. Continue to use your elevated commode seat after you have been discharged from the hospital, until cleared by the doctor (usually around 6 to 10 weeks).

6. Do not cross legs while walking, especially when turning.

7. Avoid bending past 80 degrees (touching feet, pulling up pants, picking up something off of floor, pulling up blankets while in bed, etc.).

8. Sit in a slightly reclined position—avoid leaning forward when sitting or on commode. Do not let shoulders get ahead of hips when sitting or coming to stand.

9. Avoid raising knee higher than hip when sitting in a chair.

10. Do not try to get into a bathtub for a bath, unless using a tub chair.

General Principles

1. *Going up and down stairs:*

Up—step up with uninvolved leg, keeping crutches on the step below until both feet are on the step above, then bring both crutches up on the step.

Down—place crutches on the step below, step down with the involved leg, and then with the uninvolved leg.

2. Continue to use your crutches/walker until you return to see your doctor.

3. Avoid sitting for longer than 1 hour before standing and stretching.

4. You can return to driving 6 weeks after surgery only if you have good control over the involved leg and can move your extremity from accelerator to brake with little effort.

5. Place nightstand on the same side of the bed as the uninvolved leg. Avoid twisting the trunk toward the involved side, which would be the same as turning the leg inward.

6. Try to lie flat in bed at least 15 to 30 minutes per day to prevent tightness in front part of hip.

7. If you find you have increased swelling in the involved leg after going home, try propping foot up (remembering to lean back)—if swelling persists, contact your doctor. Also contact your doctor if you develop calf tenderness. Remember that as long as there is touch weight bearing only, the muscles are not acting to pump blood up the leg, so the leg is likely to swell somewhat until full weight bearing is established. This swelling usually disappears during the night.

EXERCISE PROGRESSION

• Hip abduction: progress exercises from isometric abduction against self-resistance to Theraband wrapped around the knees. At 5 to 6 weeks, begin standing hip abduction exercises with pulleys, sports cord, or weights. Also may perform side-stepping with a sports cord around the hips, as well as lateral step-ups with a low step, if clinically safe (see Fig. 5-13).

Progress hip abduction exercises until the patient exhibits a normal gait with good abductor strength. Our progression for a postoperative cemented prosthesis with no trochanteric osteotomy generally follows the outline below.

1. Supine isometric abduction against hand or bedrail (2 or 3 days)

Continued

REHABILITATION PROTOCOL—cont'd

Total Hip Arthroplasty

EXERCISE PROGRESSION—cont'd

2. Supine abduction sliding the involved leg out and back

3. Side-lying abduction with the involved leg on top and abduction against gravity (see Fig. 7-1)

4. Standing abduction moving the leg out to side and back (Fig. 7-4)

5. Theraband (C) exercises, sports cord, and step-ups (5 to 6 weeks)

Perform prone-lying extension exercises of the hip to strengthen the gluteus maximus (Fig. 7-5). These may be performed with the knee flexed (to isolate the gluteus maximus) and with the knee extended to strengthen the hamstrings and gluteus maximus.

■ *Note: This exercise progression is slower in certain patients (see p. 320)*

- General strengthening exercises: develop endurance, cardiovascular exercise, and general strengthening of all extremities.

DISCHARGE INSTRUCTIONS

- Continue previous exercises and ambulation activities.
- Continue to observe hip precautions.
- Install elevated toilet seat in home.
- Supply walker for home.
- Review rehabilitation specific to home situation (steps, stairwells, narrow doorways, etc.).
- Ensure home physical therapy and/or home nursing care has been arranged.
- Orient family to patient's needs, abilities, and limitations, and review hip precautions with family members.
- Reiterate avoidance of driving for 6 weeks (most cars have very low seats).
- Give patient a prescription for prophylactic antibiotics that may be needed eventually for dental or urologic procedure.

■ *We use the Campbell Clinic algorithm and the Primary Total Hip Replacement Care Pathway by Cameron shown in Clinical Orthopaedic Rehabilitation. These regimens should be modified as required to fit the patient's individual clinical needs.*

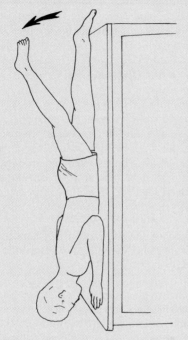

Figure 7-5 Prone-lying extension exercises of the hip are performed to strengthen the gluteus maximus. Lying prone, the patient lifts the leg 8 to 10 inches from the floor, keeping knee locked.

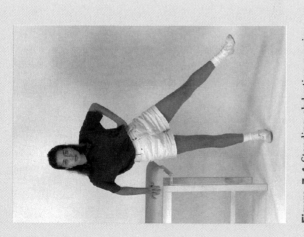

Figure 7-4 Standing abduction moving the leg out to side and back.

Managing Problems

Trendelenburg gait (weak hip abductors):

Concentrate on hip abduction exercises to strengthen abductors.

Evaluate leg-length discrepancy.

Have patient stand on involved leg while flexing opposite (uninvolved) knee 30 degrees. If opposite hip drops, have patient try to lift and hold in an effort to reeducate and work the gluteus medius muscle (hip abductor).

Flexion contracture of the hip:

AVOID placing pillows under the knee after surgery.

Walking backward helps stretch flexion contracture.

Perform the Thomas stretch test for a total of 30 stretches a day (5 stretches 6 times per day). Pull the uninvolved knee to the chest while supine. Push the involved leg into extension against the bed. This stretches the anterior capsule and hip flexors of the involved leg.

Gait Faults

Gait faults should be watched for and corrected. Chandler points out that most gait faults are either caused by or contribute to flexion deformities at the hip.

The first and most common gait fault occurs when the patient takes a large step with the involved leg and a short step with the uninvolved leg. The patient does this to avoid extension of the involved leg, which causes a stretching discomfort in the groin. The patient should be taught to concentrate on taking longer strides with the uninvolved extremity.

A second common gait fault occurs when the patient breaks the knee in late stance phase. Again, this is done to avoid extension of the hip. It is associated with flexion of the knee and early and excessive heel rise at late stance phase. The patient should be instructed to keep the heel on the ground in late stance phase.

A third common gait fault occurs when the patient flexes forward at the waist in mid and late stance. Once again the patient is attempting to avoid hip extension. To correct this, teach the patient to thrust the pelvis forward and the shoulders backward during mid and late stance phase of gait.

One additional fault, a limp, occasionally arises simply as a habit that can be difficult to break. A full-length mirror is a useful adjunct in gait training because it allows patients to observe themselves while walking toward it.

All of these gait faults are corrected with observation and teaching, as well as with increased stretching exercises to aid hip extension (e.g., Thomas test stretching).

Therapist may stretch in the Thomas test position or with the patient hanging the involved leg laterally off the table as the therapist stabilizes the pelvis and gently stretches the anterior hip structures (Fig. 7-6).

Other Important Rehabilitation Parameters:

Stair training:

> Going up stairs: step up first with the uninvolved leg, keeping crutches on the step below until both feet are on the step above, then bring both crutches up on the step.
>
> Going down stairs: place crutches on the step below, then step down with the involved leg, then with the uninvolved leg.

Restraints of home environment and activities of daily living (ADLs):

Position of Instability (Cameron)

- Posterior dislocation: flexion, adduction, and internal rotation
- Anterior dislocation: extension, adduction, and external rotation

---

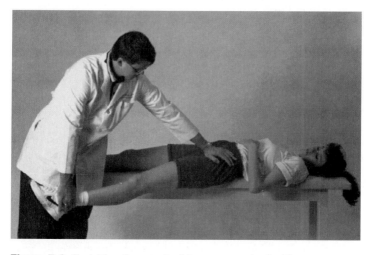

Figure 7-6 Stretching the anterior hip structures in the Thomas test position.

Assess home environment and activities of daily living for unique rehabilitation problems:

Assess home equipment needs

Assess unique barriers to mobility

Institute a home exercise program that may be realistically performed

Cane:

We also advocate the long-term use of a cane in the contralateral hand to minimize daily forces across the hip arthroplasty and, it is hoped, to prolong implant longevity (Fig. 7-7).

Stair Training

The good go up to heaven: "Good" extremity goes first upstairs.

The bad go down to hell: "Bad" or involved extremity goes first downstairs.

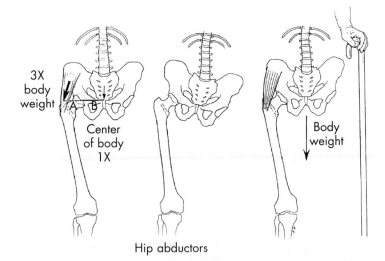

Hip abductors

Figure 7-7 The use of a cane redirects the force across the hip. Without the cane, the resultant force across the hip is about 3 times body weight, because the force of the abductors acts on the greater trochanter to offset body weight and levels the pelvis in single stance. (From Kyle RF: *Fractures of the hip.* In Gustilo RB, Kyle RF, Templeman D: *Fractures and dislocations*, St. Louis, 1993, Mosby–Year Book.)

Total Knee Arthroplasty

REHABILITATION RATIONALE

Indications for total knee arthroplasty include disabling knee pain with functional impairment and radiographic evidence of significant arthritic involvement, and failed conservative measures, including ambulatory aids (cane), nonsteroidal antiinflammatory medications (NSAIDs), and life-style modification.

Contraindications for total knee arthroplasty:

Absolute

- Recent or current joint infection—unless carrying out an infected revision
- Sepsis or systemic infection
- Neuropathic arthropathy
- Painful solid knee fusion (Painful healed knee fusions are usually due to reflex sympathetic dystrophy. Reflex sympathetic dystrophy is not helped by additional surgery.)

Relative contraindications

- Severe osteoporosis
- Debilitated poor health
- Nonfunctioning extensor mechanism
- Painless, well-functioning arthrodesis
- Significant peripheral vascular disease

GOALS OF REHABILITATION AFTER TOTAL KNEE ARTHROPLASTY

- Prevent hazards of bedrest (DVT, pulmonary embolism [PE], pressure ulcers, etc.).
- Assist with adequate and functional ROM:
    Strengthen knee musculature
    Assist patient in achieving functional independent ADLs
- Independent ambulation with an assistive device

REHABILITATION RATIONALE

Many surgeons use an identical routine, whether implants are cemented or noncemented, the rationale being that the initial fixation of noncemented femoral components is in general so good that loosening is a very uncommon occurrence. The tibial component is largely loaded in compression. The stability achieved with pegs and screws may not be adequate to prevent micromotion (which may prevent bone ingrowth of up to 100 microns). Stem fixation may reduce the micromotion to a level such that full, immediate weight bearing can be allowed. To date the literature is

Classification of Tricompartmental Total Knee Implants

Constraint

Unconstrained

Relies heavily on soft tissue integrity to provide joint stability

Rarely used in total knee arthroplasty

Semiconstrained

Most knee prostheses fall into this group

With judicious soft tissue releases and proper implant selection, flexion contractures up to 45 degrees and angular deformities up to 25 degrees can be corrected

Fully Constrained

Fully constrained in one or more planes of motion

Because of restriction of motion in one or more planes of motion, implant stresses are very high with potentially higher incidence of loosening, excessive wear, and breakage

Reserved for severe instability and severe deformity too large for semiconstrained implants.

silent on this issue. The progression of weight bearing at present, therefore, is based solely on the surgeon's discretion.

The guidelines given here are general guidelines and may have to be tailored to individual patients. Concomitant osteotomies or significant structural bone grafting should be an indication for limited weight bearing until union has been achieved. Similarly, if the bone is extremely osteoporotic, a delay in full weight bearing until the periimplant bone plate develops may be indicated.

Exposure problems requiring tibial tubercle osteotomy or a quadriceps tendon division may indicate that straight leg raising be avoided until adequate healing has been achieved, which may take 4 to 8 weeks.

PERIOPERATIVE REHABILITATION CONSIDERATIONS

Component design, fixation method, bone quality, and operative technique (osteotomy, extensor mechanism technique) will all af-

---

Fixation Method for Total Knee Implants

Cemented
Used for older, more sedentary patients

Porous Ingrowth
Theoretically, porous ingrowth fixation should not deteriorate with time (unlike cemented fixation) and is thus the ideal choice for younger or more active candidates

Hybrid Technique
Noncemented "ingrowth" femoral and patellar component with a cemented tibial component
Frequently used because of failure to achieve fixation with some of the original porous-coated tibial components as reported in the literature

---

fect perioperative rehabilitation. Implants can be posterior cruciate sacrificing, posterior cruciate sacrificing with substitution, or posterior cruciate retaining. See the box for advantages and disadvantages of these component designs.

Ninety degrees of flexion is generally considered the minimum requirement for ADLs. Those from cultures such as Japan and Korea may prefer a much greater range of movement as may the followers of Islam. Flexion of 90 degrees is generally required to descend stairs (Fox). Flexion of at least 105 degrees is required to arise easily from a low chair (Fox). Patients with less than 100 to 115 degrees of flexion preoperatively tend to increase their motion postoperatively.

Orthopaedic Knowledge Update (OKU) #4 asserts that a flexion contracture of 20 degrees or less immediately after surgery often corrects with physical therapy. Therefore, they recommend that the inability to obtain full extension intraoperatively is not an absolute indication for further bone resection, as long as attention is paid to posterior capsular release and posterior femoral osteophyte excision.

Continuous Passive Motion (CPM)

There is conflicting data on the long-term effects of continuous passive motion (CPM) on ROM, DVT, pulmonary emboli, and pain relief. Several studies have shown a shorter period of hospitalization with the use of CPM by shortening the length of time required

Rehabilitation of Patients With "Hybrid" Ingrowth Implants Versus Those With Cemented Total Knee Implants

Cemented Total Knee Arthroplasty
• Ability for weight bearing as tolerated with walker from 1 day postoperatively

"Hybrid" or Ingrowth Total Knee Arthroplasty
• TDWB only with walker for first 6 weeks
• Next 6 weeks begin crutch walking with weight bearing as tolerated

Note: Surgeon's preference may be different.

PCL—Sacrifice or Retain

Advantages of Preserving the PCL
• Potentially restores more normal knee kinematics, resulting in a more normal stair climbing ability compared to those with PCL sacrificing knees.

Disadvantages of Preserving the PCL
• Excessive rollback of the femur on the tibia if too tight
• The preoperative joint line must be reproduced.
• More difficult collateral ligament balancing.
• More difficulty in correcting large flexion contractures.

to achieve 90 degrees of flexion. However, an increased incidence of wound complications also has been reported. Reports vary on whether there is any long-term (1 year) improvement of postoperative flexion in patients receiving CPM versus those not receiving CPM.

■ *Transcutaneous oxygen tension of the skin near the incision for total knee replacement has been shown to decrease significantly after the knee is flexed more than 40 degrees. Therefore, a CPM rate of 1 cycle per minute and a maximum flexion limited to 40 degrees for the first 3 days is recommended.*

Total Knee Arthroplasty—Outline

Preoperative (Physical Therapy)
- Review transfers with patient:
  Bed-to-chair transfers
  Bathroom transfers
  Tub transfers with tub chair at home
- Teach postoperative knee exercises and give patient handout.
- Teach ambulation with assistive device (walker):
  TDWB or WBAT for total knee arthroplasty at the discretion of the surgeon.
- Review precautions:
To prevent possible dislocation, Insall recommends avoiding hamstring exercises in a sitting position when using a posterior stabilized prosthesis (cruciate sacrificing).

Inpatient Rehabilitation Goals
- 0 to 90 degrees ROM in the first 2 weeks before discharge from an inpatient (hospital or rehabilitation unit) setting
- Rapid return of quadriceps control and strength to enable patient to ambulate without knee immobilizer
- Safety during ambulation with walker and transfers
- Rapid mobilization to minimize risks of bed rest
Because of tradeoffs between early restoration of knee ROM (especially flexion) and wound stability in the early postoperative period, two separate protocols are used at the Campbell Clinic, according to surgeon preference. Both of these protocols are presented.

If a CPM unit is used, the leg seldom comes out into full extension. Such a device must be removed several times a day so that the patient can work to prevent the development of a fixed flexion deformity.

Manipulation
The ususal site of adhesions is the suprapatellar pouch. If a manipulation is to be carried out, it is better done early. An early (e.g., around 2 weeks) manipulation can be carried out with minimal force. Adhesions begin to gain in strength after this time, and a late (e.g., around 4 weeks) manipulation may require considerable force, potentially leading to complications.

REHABILITATION PROTOCOL

Total Knee Arthroplasty—"Accelerated"

Day 1
- Initiate isometric exercises (p. 344).
  Straight leg raises
  Quad sets
  Ankle pumps
- Ambulate twice a day with knee immobilizer, assistance, and walker.

■ NOTE: *Use immobilizer during ambulation until patient is able to perform 3 straight leg raises in succession out of the immobilizer.*

- Cemented prosthesis:
  WBAT with walker
- Noncemented prosthesis:
  TDWB with walker
- Transfer out of bed and into chair twice a day with leg in full extension on stool or another chair (see Fig. 5-3).
- **CPM machine:**
  Do not allow more than 40 degrees of flexion on settings until after 3 days
  Usually 1 cycle per minute

2 days through 2 weeks
- Progress 5 to 10 degrees a day as tolerated
  Do not record passive ROM measurements from CPM machine, but rather from patient because these may differ 5 to 10 degrees.
- Initiate active ROM and active-assisted ROM exercises (pp. 344 and 345).
- During sleep, replace the knee immobilizer and place a pillow under the ankle to help knee extension.
- Proceed with Campbell Clinic total knee protocol (see *Clinical Orthopaedic Rehabilitation*).
- Continue isometric exercises throughout rehabilitation.
- Use vastus medialis oblique (VMO) biofeedback if patient is having difficulty with quadriceps strengthening or control (see Fig. 5-2).

2 days through 2 weeks —cont'd	• Begin gentle passive ROM exercises for knee ROM:
	  Knee extension (Fig. 7-8)
	  Knee flexion
	  Heel slides
	  Wall slides
	• Begin patellar mobilization techniques when incision stable (postoperative day 3 to 5) to avoid contracture (see Fig. 5-10).
		• Perform active hip abduction and adduction exercises.
		• Continue active and active-assisted knee ROM exercises.
		• Continue and progress these exercises until 6 weeks after surgery. Give home exercises with outpatient physical therapist following patient 2 to 3 times per week.
		• Provide discharge instructions. Plan discharge when ROM of involved knee is from 0 to 90 degrees and patient can independently execute transfers and ambulation.

10 days through 3 weeks		• Discharge instructions (10 days to 3 weeks after surgery) • Plan discharge when 0-90 degrees ROM and independent in transfers and ambulation • Continue previous exercises. • Continue use of walker until otherwise instructed by physician.

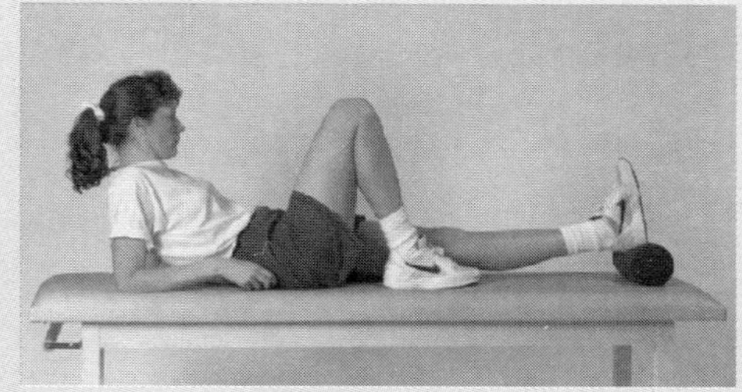

Figure 7-8 Passive extension exercises for knee. Place towel under foot. Slow, sustained push with hands downward on quadriceps.

Continued

REHABILITATION PROTOCOL—cont'd

Total Knee Arthroplasty—"Accelerated"

10 days to 3 weeks —cont'd	• Ensure that home physical therapy and/or home nursing care has been arranged.
	• Prescribe prophylactic antibiotics for possible eventual dental or urologic procedures.
	• Do not permit driving for 4 to 6 weeks.
	• Provide walker for home and equipment/supplies as needed.
	• Orient family to patient's needs, abilities, and limitations.
	• Review tub transfers:
	  Many patients lack sufficient strength, ROM, or agility to step over tub for showering
	  Place tub chair as far back in tub as possible, facing the faucets. Patient backs up to the tub, sits on the chair, and then lifts the leg over.
	  Tub mats and nonslip stickers for tub-floor traction also are recommended.

6 weeks	• Begin weight bearing as tolerated with ambulatory aid, if not already.
	• Perform wall slides; progress to lunges (see Figs. 5-1 and 5-14).
	• Perform quadriceps dips or step-ups.
	• Begin closed-chain knee exercises on total gym and progress over 4 to 5 weeks:
	  Bilateral lower extremities
	  Single leg exercises (see Fig. 5-11)
	  Incline
	• Progress stationary bicycling.
	• Perform lap-stool exercises (hamstring strengthening).
	• Cone walking: progress from 4- to 6- to 8-inch cones.
	• Use McConnell taping of patella to unload patellofemoral stress if patellofemoral symptoms occur with exercise.
	• Continue home physical therapy exercises.

REHABILITATION PROTOCOL (#2)

Total Knee Arthroplasty CAMPBELL CLINIC

This protocol usually is followed by patients who have a high likelihood of delayed or impaired wound healing (chronic steroid use, diabetes mellitus, etc.).

Day 1
- Begin isometric exercises (see p. 344).
  Ankle pumps
- ■ CPM is not used.
- Ambulate twice a day with knee immobilizer, walker, and assistance.

3 days
- Begin active ROM exercises and active-assisted ROM exercises (right hand column) if wound is clean and dry.
- Ambulate without knee immobilizer when patient is able to perform 3 straight leg raises in succession without immobilizer.

- Initiate passive ROM exercises on day 3 or 4 for knee flexion and extension.
- Proceed with Campbell Clinic protocol (see *Clinical Orthopaedic Rehabilitation*).

6 weeks
- Initiate the exercises listed in the accelerated protocol (see p. 342).
- ■ Note: *The difference between these two protocols is the avoidance of CPM in patients with possible wound healing problems in this protocol.*

Continued

REHABILITATION PROTOCOL (#2)—cont'd

Total Knee Arthroplasty   CAMPBELL CLINIC

Postoperative Exercise Program Total Knee Replacement—cont'd

Quadriceps sets	• Tighten knees, pushing them down into the bed, feeling thigh tighten. Hold for 5 seconds, then relax. • ____ sets of ____. • Repeat session ____ times a day.
Straight leg raises	• Lie on back keeping knee straight and foot pointed upward. • Lift the leg slowly and then return to starting position. • ____ sets of ____. • Repeat ____ times a day.
Ankle pumps	• Move foot up and hold, move foot down and hold.
Knee flexion (active-assisted ROM)	• ____ sets of ____. • Repeat ____ times a day. • Sitting, slide foot backward as far as possible and then plant operated foot on ground. • While foot is planted slide knee out over foot and count to 10. • ____ sets of ____. • Repeat ____ times a day.
Knee flexion (active-assisted ROM)	• Sitting, gently lower leg to fully flexed position. • Gently push involved leg back with the good leg until you feel a good stretch. • ____ sets of ____. • Repeat session ____ times a day.

Passive knee extension	• Sit with knee propped on a stool so that the knee tends to sag.
	• Press hands down on thigh and hold for a count of 10.
	• _____ sets of _____.
	• Repeat session _____ times a day.
Knee flexion to extension (active ROM)	• Sit with foot as far back as possible, then move foot outward and upward, and then hold for a count of 5.
	• _____ sets of _____.
	• Repeat session _____ times a day.
Hamstring curls (active ROM)	• Standing, raise foot up behind you and hold for a count of 3.
	• _____ sets of _____.
	• Repeat session _____ times a day.
Additional exercises:	_____
	_____
	_____
	_____
	• At 6 weeks initiate the exercises listed in accelerated protocol. The difference between these two protocols is avoidance of CPM in patients with possible wound healing problems in this protocol.

Management of Rehabilitation Problems

Recalcitrant Flexion Contracture (Difficulty Obtaining Full Knee Extension)

- Initiate backwards walking.
- Eccentric extension:
  Therapist passively extends the leg and then holds the leg as the patient attempts to lower it slowly.
- With the patient standing, flex and extend the involved knee. Sports cord or rubber bands can be used for resistance.
- Use electrical stimulation and VMO biofeedback for muscle re-education if problem is active extension.
- Perform passive extension with the patient lying prone with the knee off the table, with and without weight placed across the ankle (see Fig. 5-10, *B*). This should be avoided if contraindicated by the PCL status of the arthroplasty.
- Passive extension also is performed with a towel roll placed under the ankle and the patient pushing downward on the femur (or with weight on top of the femur). (See Fig. 5-10, *A*.)

Delayed Knee Flexion

- Passive stretching into flexion by therapist.
- Wall slides for gravity assistance.
- Stationary bicycle:
  If patient lacks enough motion to bicycle with saddle high, then begin cycling backwards, then forward, until they are able to make a revolution. Typically, this can be done first in a backward fashion.

Recommended Long-Term Activities After Total Joint Replacement

DeAndrade developed an evaluation scale of the activities for patients with total joint replacements. Stress on the replacement should be minimized to avoid excessive wear and tear that would reduce the longevity of the implant. Intensity of the exercise should be adjusted so that it is painless, but still promotes cardiovascular fitness. Running and jumping should be avoided, and shoes should be well cushioned in the heel and insole. Joints should not be placed at the extremes of motion. Activity time should be built up gradually, with frequent rest periods between activity periods. Correct use of walking aids is encouraged to minimize stress on the joint replacement. The first long-term activity undertaken should be walking (Table 7-1).

TABLE 7-1 **Recommended Long-Term Activities After Total Replacement of the Hip or Knee (DeAndrade)**

Very Good, Highly Recommended	Good, Recommended	Needs Some Skill, Prior Significant Expertise	With Care, Ask Your Doctor	AVOID
Stationary bicycling	Bowling	Bicycling (street)	Aerobic exercise	Baseball
Ballroom dancing	Fencing	Canoeing	Calisthenics	Basketball
Square dancing	Rowing	Horseback riding	Jazz dancing	Football
Golf	Speed walking	Rock climbing		Softball
Stationary (Nordic-Track) skiing	Table tennis	Inline skating		Handball
Swimming	Cross-country skiing	Nautilus exercises		Jogging
Walking				Racquetball/squash
		Ice skating	Downhill skiing	Lacrosse
			Tennis—doubles	Soccer
Weight-lifting			Step machines (for patients with hip replacements; not for those with knee replacements)	Tennis—singles
				Volleyball

CHAPTER EIGHT

Low Back Disorders

ARTHUR H. WHITE, MD
S. BRENT BROTZMAN, MD

Rehabilitation Rationale

Low back disability appears to have dramatically increased in Western society over the last 30 years. Waddell concluded, however, that this is not indicative of an increase in injuries or in the occurrence of low back pain, but rather of an increase in work loss, sick certification, compensation, and long-term disability award.

ACUTE BACK PAIN

Acute back pain is common, affecting between 70% and 85% of adults at some point in their lives. Back complaints are second only to upper respiratory conditions as a cause of work absenteeism. An estimated 1.3 billion days a year are lost from work because of back pain. The usual onset of low back pain is in the third decade of life, with the peak prevalence during the fifth decade.

Some risk factors have become evident. Nondisabling low back pain is three times more common in pregnant women than in their nonparous counterparts. Cigarette smoking has been found to be a possible risk factor for low back pain, as well as low back pain with concomitant sciatica due to lumbar disc herniation. Occupational risk factors associated with an increased risk of developing acute low back pain or delayed recovery include (1) employees' perceptions of their jobs as boring, dissatisfying, or repetitious, (2) an unpleasant or noisy work environment, (3) perception of poor social support in the work environment with regard to employer/ employee interaction, and (4) the employer's perception of the employee as less competent.

Eighty percent to 90% of patients with acute low back pain episodes recover in about 6 weeks, regardless of the administration or type of treatment. Nearly 60% of patients return to work within 1 week. In patients whose symptoms of chronic back pain result in continued work loss, the likelihood of returning to work 6 months after an episode is 50%, by 1 year 20%, and at 2 years the probability of return approaches 0%. The return-to-work rate is significantly diminished with the presence of a lawyer or threatened legal action. The rate of recurrence after an acute low back pain episode ranges from 40% to 85%.

INTRADISCAL PRESSURE

Response to *disc pressure* is an important indication of an acute herniated disc (HNP). Patients with HNP are typically most comfortable in a recumbent position, less comfortable standing, and least comfortable sitting. Nachemson's intradiscal pressure studies in living subjects suggest the reason for this: intradiscal pressure increases progressively from supine, standing, and sitting postures. Side-lying also has a notable increase in intradiscal pressure.

Nachemson's studies showed that active extension of the back in the prone position increases intradiscal pressure (Fig. 8-1), and

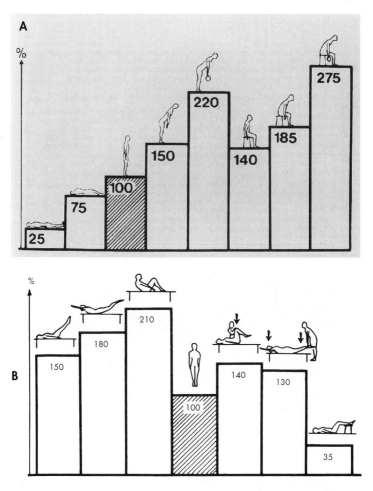

Figure 8-1 **A,** Relative change in pressure (or load) in the third lumbar disc in various positions in living subjects. **B,** Relative change in pressure (or load) in the third lumbar disc in various muscle-strengthening exercises in living subjects. (From Nachemson A: *The lumbar spine, an orthopaedic challenge, Spine* 1:59, 1976.)

McKenzie emphasizes *passive* back extension in his exercise regimen (Fig. 8-2). Extension allows the viscoelastic disc to "milk forward" (Fig. 8-3, *B*), but prevents any free (extruded) disc fragment from migrating anteriorly (Fig. 8-3, *D*). Increased nerve-root pressure by constriction at the intervertebral foramen may increase radicular pain. Any radicular pain increase with extension is a contraindication to extension therapy, but an initial increase in localized back pain only with extension therapy is not a contraindication and, in fact, may be expected.

Williams flexion exercises have been used for both low back pain and HNP (Fig. 8-4). Nachemson's demonstration that Williams first exercise increased intradiscal pressure to 210% over standing appears to contradict the use of these exercises in patients with HNP. In fact, three of the six exercises in the Williams regimen were found to increase intradiscal pressures significantly.

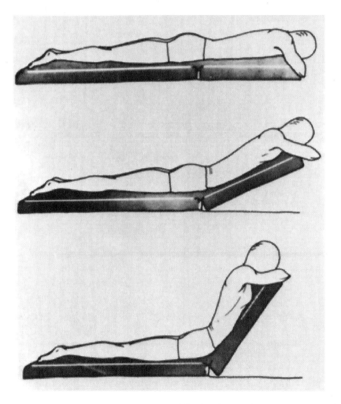

Figure 8-2 Passive extension using table. (Redrawn from McKenzie RA: *The lumbar spine: mechanical diagnosis in therapy,* Waidanae, NZ, 1981, Spinal.)

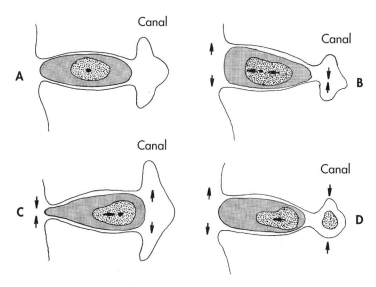

Figure 8-3 A, The nucleus pulposus with spine in neutral. **B,** The nucleus pulposus with the spine in extension. **C,** The nucleus pulposus with the spine in flexion. **D,** Extension with extruded fragment. The fragment cannot return through the incompetent anulus fibrosus and, as a consequence, must share the narrowed foramen with nerve root, increasing symptoms. (Redrawn from McKenzie RA: *The lumbar spine: mechanical diagnosis in therapy,* Waidanae, NZ, 1981, Spinal.)

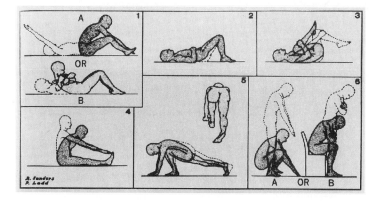

Figure 8-4 Williams postural exercises. (From Williams PC: *The lumbosacral spine, emphasizing conservative management,* New York, 1965, McGraw-Hill.)

Treatment

The goals of treatment of acute low back pain are shown in the box. Most patients with low back pain can be successfully treated with conservative measures. The most commonly used treatment methods are bed rest and exercise.

BED REST

Bed rest is the most frequently used treatment for low back pain. The traditional rationale for bed rest is twofold: (1) many patients with mechanical low back pain, as well as those with HNP, report symptomatic relief in the supine position, and (2) measurements indicate that intradiscal pressure is minimized in the supine position. However, nearly 50% of patients with back pain report only minimal relief with bed rest, and intradiscal pressure rises to 75% of that in the standing position when patients simply roll onto their side.

Comparison of 2 days of bed rest to 7 days of bed rest in outpatient-clinic patients with acute low back pain revealed equally prompt pain resolution and return of function, but those given the shorter bed rest recommendation returned to work 45% sooner (3.1 versus 5.6 days). Thus, it appears that in patients with no neuromotor deficits, 2 days of bed rest are as effective as longer periods. A similar study compared 4 days of bed rest to no bed rest in 270 patients. Those with no bed rest returned to their usual activities 42% faster than those with 4 days of bed rest. Gilbert et al. found no statistically significant differences between bed rest, exercise, and no treatment, although the results tended to favor early mobilization.

Goals of Treatment of Acute Low Back Pain

- Alleviate pain
- Promote healing of injured tissue
- Relieve muscle spasm
- Restore normal range of motion (ROM), spinal mechanics, and muscle function
- Educate patient to prevent further episodes
- Return patient to activities of daily living/workplace

■ *Studies suggest that although bed rest may provide some symptomatic relief for patients with acute low back pain, a brief period (if any) should be sufficient. Bed rest does not appear to alter the natural history of recovery.*

Bed rest also has medical and social side effects. According to Deyo, these may include perception of severe illness (even myocardial infarction does not require a week of strict bed rest); economic loss (absenteeism is strongly related to bed rest); muscle atrophy (1% to 1.5% per day); cardiopulmonary deconditioning (15% in 10 days); and acute complications such as thromboembolism, bone mineral loss, hypercalcemia, and hypercalciuria. To prevent deconditioning, many experts now recommend at least a brief daily ambulation for patients with HNP, with or without neurologic deficit, after 3 days of bed rest. Several studies have demonstrated improved disc nutrition with motion.

Compliance is also a problem. Most patients sit to read or watch television, raising intradiscal pressure to a level higher than that in a standing position.

EXERCISE PROGRAMS

Several exercise programs have been developed for acute low back pain. These include those designed by McKenzie (mainly extension exercises), Williams, Aston, Heller, and Feldenkreis, and other lumbar stabilization programs, stretching regimens, and aerobic conditioning programs.

McKenzie Technique

The McKenzie technique is one of the most popular of the many conservative care programs. It is a method of diagnosis and treatment based on movement patterns of the spine. For any spinal condition, certain movements aggravate the pain and other movements relieve the pain. Because the McKenzie method works best for acute back pain that responds to lumbar extension, mobilization, and exercises, the technique has been erroneously labeled an extension exercise program. McKenzie, in fact, advocates position and movement patterns, flexion or extension, that best relieve the patient's symptoms.

McKenzie's method is complex and much has been written explaining its theoretical basis. In his text, *The Lumbar Spine: Mechanical Diagnosis and Therapy,* he classifies low back pain based on spinal movement patterns, positions, and pain responses, and describes a postural syndrome, derangement, and dysfunction. Each classification has a specific treatment that includes education and some form of postural correction. A basic explanation of the method is as follows. Some stages of the lumbar degenerative cascade create symptoms because of pathoanatomic abnormalities, which can be positively altered by spinal positioning. This hypothesis has led to several forms of spinal manipulation, including chiropractic and osteopathy. The McKenzie technique is a more passive form of spinal manipulation in which the patient produces the motion, position, and forces that improve the condition. Examples of pathoanatomic alterations include a tear in the anulus and acute facet arthritis. Repeated lumbar extension may reduce edema and nuclear migration in an anular tear or may realign a facet joint in such a way as to reduce inflammation and painful stimuli. Through trial and error, the position and exercise program that best relieve the patient's symptoms can be found.

Cyclic ROM exercises (usually in passive extension) are the cornerstone of the McKenzie program. These repetitive exercises "centralize" pain, and certain postures prevent end-range stress. Lumbar flexion exercises may be added later, when the patient has full spinal ROM.

Treatment is based on evaluation of pain location and maneuvers that change the pain location from referred to centralized. Once identified, the direction of exercise and movement (such as extension) is used for treatment. Centralization, as McKenzie uses the term, refers to a rapid change in perceived location of pain from a distal or peripheral location to a proximal or central one. Donelson et al. reported centralization of asymmetric or radiating pain in 87% of patients during the first 48 hours of care.

For a movement to eventually centralize pain, it must be performed repetitively, because the initial movement often aggravates or intensifies the pain. Centralization also occurs more rapidly if the initial movements are performed passively to end range. Centralization most frequently occurs as a result of extension movement, occasionally from lateral movements, and only rarely with flexion.

McKenzie reported that 98% of patients with symptoms for less than 4 weeks who experienced centralization during their initial assessment had excellent or good results; 77% of patients with subacute symptoms (4 to 12 weeks) had excellent or good results if their pain centralized initially.

The great value of this program is that it gives patients an understanding of their condition and responsibility for maintaining proper alignment and function. Disadvantages are that the program requires active, willing participation of the patient, who must have the ability to centralize the pain; better results are obtained for patients with acute pain than for those with chronic pain, and the complex regimen requires a therapist trained in McKenzie's techniques to obtain the best results.

REHABILITATION PROTOCOL

Acute Low Back Pain MC KENZIE

McKenzie recommends implementation of this protocol by a therapist with specialized training in the McKenzie method to ensure proper recognition and correct implementation of treatment in response to the patient's clinical relief derived from specific maneuvers. To determine which exercises produce centralization, the physical therapist tests the patient with a standardized series of lumbar movements, such as flexion, extension, lateral bending, rotation, and side-gliding (a combination of lateral bending and rotation). Once the therapist identifies the movement (usually extension or lateral bending) that decreases peripheral symptoms, the patient is taught to perform an individualized exercise program in that direction of movement. The movement is performed repetitively to the passive end range. Maneuvers that "peripheralize" or exacerbate symptoms are discontinued.

Repeat End-Range Movements While Standing

Back bending (extension) (Fig. 8-5):
The patient stands upright with feet slightly apart (*A*). Place the hands on the small of the back with fingers pointing backward. The patient then bends backward (from the waist) as far as possible, using the hands as a fulcrum (*B*). Keep the knees straight. Hold this position for 1 to 2 seconds, then the patient returns to the starting position. This exercise incorporates the effect of gravity because it is performed in an upright position.

- Side gliding (Fig. 8-6),
- Forward bending (lumbar flexion)

Continued

REHABILITATION PROTOCOL—cont'd

Acute Low Back Pain   MC KENZIE

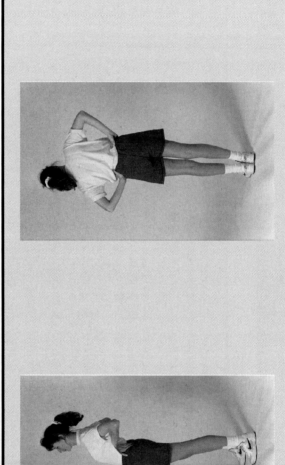

Figure 8-5 Extension in a standing posture.

Figure 8-6 Side-gliding.

Recumbent End-Range Movements

- Passive extension while prone (Fig. 8-7):

  In this exercise, the patient lies face down, with hands positioned under the shoulders (A), then pushes up by slowly extending the elbows (B) while keeping the pelvis, hips, and legs relaxed (this allows the back to sag). Maintain this position for 1 to 2 seconds, then the patient slowly lowers the upper body to the floor. This exercise eliminates the loading effects of gravity because it is performed prone.

- Knees-to-chest while supine (Fig. 8-8):

  The patient lies supine, with knees flexed and feet flat on the floor or bed (A). Patient places the hands around the knees (B) and slowly pulls both knees up toward the chest as far as possible (C). This position is maintained for 1 to 2 seconds, then the patient slowly lowers the feet back to the starting position. The patient must not raise the head while performing this exercise or straighten the legs while lowering them.

- Prone lateral shifting of hips off midline (Fig. 8-9) (patients with unilateral symptoms):

  The patient lies face down, arms at sides (A), moves hips away from the side of pain and maintains this position for a few seconds (B). With the hips off center, the patient then places the elbows under the shoulders and leans on the forearms (C and D); the patient relaxes in this position for 3 or 4 minutes. The patient can then perform the maneuver "extension while lying prone," keeping the hips off center

- Flexion while sitting (Fig. 8-10):

  The patient sits on the edge of a steady chair or stool, with legs apart and hands resting on knees (A). The patient bends forward from the waist to touch the floor with the hands. The patient holds this position for 1 to 2 seconds and then slowly returns to upright. Once able to bend forward comfortably, the patient can hold onto the ankles and pull self further down (B).

Continued

REHABILITATION PROTOCOL—cont'd

Acute Low Back Pain   MC KENZIE

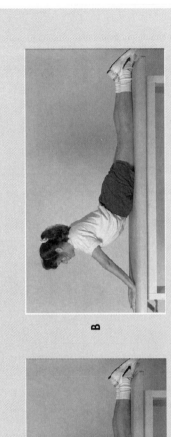

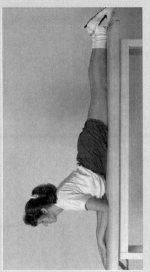

Figure 8-7 Passive extension while prone.

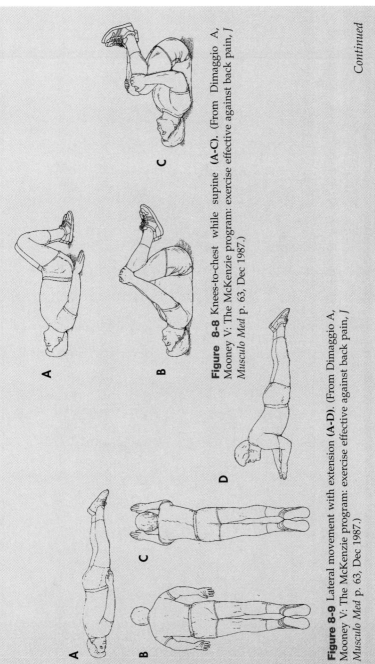

Figure 8-8 Knees-to-chest while supine **(A-C)**. (From Dimaggio A, Mooney V: The McKenzie program: exercise effective against back pain, *J Musculo Med* p. 63, Dec 1987.)

Figure 8-9 Lateral movement with extension **(A-D)**. (From Dimaggio A, Mooney V: The McKenzie program: exercise effective against back pain, *J Musculo Med* p. 63, Dec 1987.)

Continued

REHABILITATION PROTOCOL—cont'd

Acute Low Back Pain MC KENZIE

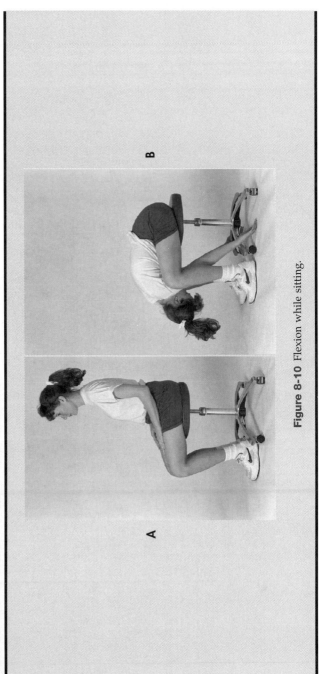

Figure 8-10 Flexion while sitting.

Each movement is taken to its end range repetitively as long as distal pain continues to diminish. McKenzie stresses the importance of taking the movements to the end range permitted by the patient to accurately observe changes in the pain pattern. If distal symptoms worsen, that specific movement is discontinued. Pain location from these maneuvers are carefully observed and recorded.

Based on the clinical response to centralization, the patient is taught to perform home spinal exercises in that direction of movement (usually extension). For example, for a patient with acute pain, the self-care exercise program may include prone extension for a few seconds at a time, with sets of 10 repetitions performed every hour or two. The patient is also taught modified resting positions (for sitting, standing, and lying) and work postures that will maintain centralization and avoid peripheralization.

Most patients have centralization of pain in the first 2 days or sooner. Treatment outcomes in "centralizers" are typically good.

McKenzie classified lumbar movements that have the potential to centralize symptoms into extension, flexion, lateral bending, rotation, and side-gliding (combination of lateral bending and rotation). These may be used individually or in combination to diminish the peripheral pain. Gravity-elimination (prone) versus gravity-assisted (standing) symptom reduction further increases the number of lumbar-movement combinations that the therapist must understand and possibly use in an effort to centralize symptoms. The result is that more than 40 different exercise regimens are available, and application of the appropriate regimen may require complex customization.

Williams Flexion Exercises (see Fig. 8-4)
The goals of this isometric flexion regimen, developed in the 1930s, are to (1) widen the intervertebral foramina and facet joint to reduce nerve compression, (2) stretch hip flexors and back extensors, (3) strengthen abdominal and gluteal muscles, and (4) reduce "posterior fixation" of the lumbosacral junction. A concern with this method is that certain flexion maneuvers increase intradiscal pressure, possibly aggravating herniated or bulging discs. According to Nachemson, Williams' first exercise increases intradiscal pressure to 210% over that in a standing posture. Three of the six exercises increase intradiscal pressure, and these three are contraindicated for patients with acute herniated disc.

Lumbar Stabilization Program
There is no evidence that early return to activity increases the likelihood of recurrences. On the contrary, physically fit individuals have fewer and shorter attacks of low back pain and are more tol-

erant of pain. With a better understanding of spinal biomechanics, specific activities and positions that increase loads on the spine can be avoided. Numerous studies have shown that patients with low back pain can perform selected activities almost normally without increasing pain. Body mechanics that avoid painful positions are called cautious or preventative body mechanics. Body mechanics that attempt to overcome the condition with muscular effort and knowledge of body positions has led to the field of stabilization training.

The main goal of the lumbar stabilization program is to build musculature that stabilizes the torso, with co-contraction of abdominal muscles to provide a corseting effect on the lumbar spine. This concept is centered on the assumption that an injured lumbar motion segment may create a weak link in the kinetic chain, with subsequent predisposition to reinjury. This program is used in conjunction with other methods aimed at controlling acute pain (such as nonsteroidal antiinflammatory medication). Emphasis is on positioning the spine in a nonpainful orientation, termed the *neutral spine*. Stretching and ROM exercises are then completed daily in this configuration. Supervision by an appropriately oriented trainer is advised.

The *second phase* of treatment consists of active joint mobilization methods, including extension exercises in prone and standing positions, and alternating midrange flexion extension in a four-point stance. Simple curl-ups for abdominal muscle strengthening is progressed to dynamic abdominal raising. This includes "dead bug" exercises, using alternate arm and leg movements while supine. Diagonal curl-ups and incline board work are performed.

Progression to aerobic exercise, exercise with a ball, and weight training may be added (see box on p. 365). The program endpoint is determined by *maximal functional improvement*, the point beyond which no further improvement in function will result from additional exercise.

Exercise Training in the Lumbar Stabilization Program

Soft Tissue Flexibility
- Hamstring musculotendinous unit
- Quadriceps musculotendinous unit
- Iliopsoas musculotendinous unit
- Gastrocnemius-soleus musculotendinous unit
- External and internal hip rotators

Joint Mobility
- Lumbar spine segmental mobility
  Extension
  Flexion (unloaded)
- Hip range of motion
- Thoracic segmental mobility

Stabilization Program
- Finding neutral position
  Standing
  Sitting
  Jumping
  Prone
- Prone gluteal squeezes
  With arm raises
  With alternate arm raises
  With leg raises
  With alternate leg raises
  With arm and leg raises
  With alternate arm and leg raises
- Supine pelvic bracing
- Bridging progression
  Basic position
    One leg raised with ankle weights
    Stepping
    Balance on gym ball

Stabilization Program—cont'd
- Quadruped
  With alternating arm and leg movements
- Kneeling stabilization
  Double knee
  Single knee
  Lunges, with and without weight
- Wall-slide quadriceps strengthening
- Position transition with postural control
  Abdominal program
    Curl-ups
    Dead bug, supported and unsupported
    Diagonal curl-ups
    Diagonal curl-ups on incline board
    Straight leg lowering
  Gym program
    Latissimus pull-downs
    Angled leg press
    Lunges
    Hyperextension bench
    General upper body weight exercises
  Aerobic program
    Progressive walking
    Swimming
    Stationary bicycling
    Cross-country ski machine
    Running
      Initially supervised on a treadmill

From Frymoyer JW: *The adult spine: principles and practice,* New York, 1991, Raven Press.

REHABILITATION PROTOCOL

Acute, Mechanical Lower Lumbar Pain

Indications
- Symptoms of less than 6 weeks' duration
- Prior examination and evaluation to correctly diagnose mechanical low back pain and rule out other etiology

Bed rest
- We do not recommend bed rest (p. 325). For the occasional patient who has had success with this type of treatment and is adamant about using it, we recommend only 2 days of supine (not lying on the side) bed-rest.

Medication
- Give nonsteroidal antiinflammatory medication unless contraindicated. Discuss the risks, warning signs, and possible complications with the patient.
- Muscle-relaxant medications may be beneficial, but their use should be strictly time limited (typically 1 week).

Exercise
- Encourage early ambulation to limit muscular and cardiovascular deconditioning.
- Restrict (limited duty) from lifting, climbing, squatting, strenuous physical activity during the initial acute pain period.
- Institute the McKenzie back exercise program if available (see p. 326). Some physicians prefer the Williams flexion exercise regimen.
- After the acute pain has subsided (typically within 2 weeks), begin further aerobic conditioning in an effort to improve spine, abdominal, and lower extremity muscular endurance.
- Avoid exercise that places major torsion or flexion forces on the spine (such as rowing). Can use swimming, stationary bicycling, and walking.
- Exercise sessions should be at least 20 minutes per session with 3 or more weekly sessions.

Education	• The patient receives instruction on avoiding movements and postures associated with back injury (Fig. 8-11):
	AVOID: Frequent lifting (25 times/day)
	Twisting while lifting
	Heavy lifting (11.3 kg or more)
	Improper static postures
	Forward bending and twisting of the trunk
	Muscle fatigue
	■ *The most deleterious of these motions appears to be simultaneous twisting and forward bending of the trunk. Kelsey et al. report a sixfold increase in back injuries as a result of this motion.*
	• Discuss manual material handling methods, including maintaining the load close to the body and avoiding twisting motions.
	• No scientific evidence supports the assertion that those in poor physical condition are prone to back injury. Despite this, training in strength and fitness should be encouraged, with emphasis on aerobic capacity, endurance, flexibility, musculoskeletal strength, and cardiovascular fitness. The patient may

be progressed to a lumbar stabilization program (see p. 365).

Life-style

• Encourage eating-habit modification and proper dieting. Deyo reported that individuals in upper fifth quintile of weight are at greater risk for back pain.

• The effect of cigarette smoke on intervertebral disc metabolism remains unclear. Tobacco-use studies are varied in their findings with regard to the effect of tobacco on acute back pain. One study revealed no relationship, whereas another showed predictive value for future disability in a group of healthy subjects.

Back school

• Formalized back education programs that train patients in manual materials handling, ergonomics, and stress management have had varying results. Back school should be considered for patients whose work environment points to possible benefit from such training.

Rehabilitation After Disc (HNP) Surgery

General Principles of Rehabilitation After Disc Surgery

Postoperative education and physical and psychologic training are major keys to a successful rehabilitation program.

The patient should progress into safe functional activities as rapidly as pain allows.

Therapists and trainers should be used before and after surgery to assure that the patient is using safe body mechanics during return to normal activities.

A rehabilitation plan should be developed before surgery, and the patient should be committed to follow the plan after surgery.

Before surgery, the patient should be advanced to the highest level of rehabilitation possible within the limits of pain and disease process.

After surgery, the patient should be expected to accomplish reasonable goals commensurate with the underlying condition, the surgery performed, and the general physical and psychologic resources.

Postoperative pain should be controlled to allow rehabilitation.

Patients with chronic pain or psychosocial involvement that inhibits rehabilitation should be placed in a functional restoration or chronic program.

REHABILITATION PROTOCOL

Disc Surgery

In hospital
- Generally, encourage walking on the first day after surgery.
- Reinstitute isometric abdominal and lower extremity exercises.
- Minimize sitting to lower intradiscal pressure (p. 351).
- Progressively increase walking.
- When the patient is walking comfortably and pain medication is minimal, the patient may be discharged from the hospital.

At home
- As strength increases, begin gentle isotonic leg exercises.
- Allow increased sitting after the fourth week.
- Prohibit lifting, bending, and stooping for 6 weeks, and gradually progress after the sixth week.
- Do not allow long trips for 3 months.

- Increase lower extremity strength from the eighth to twelfth weeks.

Return to work
- Allow patients with jobs requiring much walking without lifting to return to work within 4 weeks.
- In general, allow patients with jobs requiring prolonged sitting to return within 6 to 8 weeks provided minimal lifting is required.
- Heavy laborers return to modified duty in approximately 12 weeks. Patients with jobs that require exceptionally heavy manual labor may have to permanently modify their occupation or seek an occupation with lighter work loads.
- Keeping patients out of work for more than 3 months rarely improves pain relief or recovery.

Index

Minisquat, 197
Mobilization
  in flexor tendon injury
    early motion, 9-10
    noncompliant patient, 13-14
    repair of flexor pollicis longus of
      thumb, 15-21
    patellar, 209
Modified Bröstrom ankle ligament
    reconstruction, 262
Modified Delee protocol, 295
Modified DeMaio and Drez protocol,
    314-315
Modified Duran protocol
  in flexor tendon injury, 4-10
  in two-stage reconstruction for
    delayed tendon repair, 23
Modified early motion program, 11-12
Modified Hamilton protocol, 277-279
Modified Jackson protocol, 269-274
Modified Lane protocol, 275-276
Monitoring in hand replantation, 48
Müller classification of distal femoral
    fracture, 167

N

Nachemson intradiscal pressure
    studies, 350-352
Nail dynamization, 150
Nail fixation of femoral shaft fracture,
    163
Nerve compression syndromes, 35-39
Nerve injury of hand, 40-45
Nerve palsies, splinting for, 40-41
Neutral spine, 364
Nitz and Shelbourne protocol, 200-201,
    215-224
Noncemented total hip, 320
Nondisplaced extraarticular phalangeal
    fracture, 54
Nondisplaced metacarpal fracture, 59
Nondisplaced scaphoid fracture, 61
Nonsteroidal antiinflammatory drugs
  in acute, mechanical lower lumbar
    pain, 366
  in de Quervain's tenosynovitis, 33
  in patellofemoral disorders, 226, 248
  in turf toe, 305
Nucleus pulposus, 353

O

Ober's test, 234, 247
Open basket weave taping for ankle
    injury, 264, 265
Open fracture
  Gustilo-Anderson classification of,
    148-150

Open fracture—cont'd
  tibial, 180, 184-185
Open kinetic chain exercises
  in anterior cruciate ligament
    reconstruction, 196-198
  in lower extremity fracture, 152-153
  patellofemoral pain and, 226
Open reduction
  in ankle fracture, 283-288
  in avulsion fracture of finger, 56
  in bony mallet deformity, 24
  in femoral neck fracture, 154
  in Rolando fracture, 58
  in scaphoid fracture, 61
Open release in carpal tunnel
    syndrome, 36
Orthotics
  in ankle sprain, 272-274
  to prevent turf toe, 301-302
Osgood-Schlatter disease, 257
Osteotomy of femur, 320
Outrigger splint, 41

P

Pain
  acute low back, 350, 366-367
  after anterior cruciate ligament
    reconstruction, 226
  in hand replantation, 48
  in iliotibial band friction syndrome,
    235
Painful arc sign, 289
Palmer treatment algorithm, 66-67
Passive extension exercises
  in dorsal blocking splint, 5
  for low back pain, 352
  in McKenzie technique, 359, 360
  in repair of flexor pollicis longus of
    thumb, 16-17
Passive flexion exercises
  after anterior cruciate ligament
    reconstruction, 207
  in dorsal blocking splint, 5
  in repair of flexor pollicis longus of
    thumb, 16-17
Passive patellar tilt test, 245-246
Patella
  dislocation of, 172-174
  fracture of, 169-171
  function and mechanics of, 241-242
  mobilization to avoid contracture,
    209
Patellar glide test, 246-247
Patellar tendonitis, 226
Patellar tilt and subluxation, 241
Patellectomy, 169